WHAT'S MISSING FROM MEDICINE

WHAT'S MISSING FROM MEDICINE

Six Lifestyle Changes to
OVERCOME CHRONIC ILLNESS

≈

SARAY STANCIC, MD
Foreword by Dean Ornish, MD

Hierophantpublishing

Cover design by Emma Smith
Cover photo by Emily Pellecchia
Illustrations by Nusrat Priya and Frame25 Productions
Print book interior design by Frame25 Productions

If you are unable to order this book from your local bookseller, you may order directly from the publisher.

Hierophant Publishing
8301 Broadway, Suite 219
San Antonio, TX 78209
www.hierophantpublishing.com

Library of Congress Control Number: 2020944801
ISBN: 978-1-950253-06-7

10 9 8 7 6 5 4 3 2 1

*For my husband, Ralph Pellecchia, whose unwavering love
has emboldened me to persevere and overcome adversity. I love you
and thank you for the miraculous gifts, our Emily and Nicholas.*

I have an almost complete disregard of precedent, and a faith in the possibility of something better. It irritates me to be told how things have always been done. I defy the tyranny of precedent. I go for anything new that might improve the past.
—Clara Barton

Contents

Foreword

It's my pleasure to write this foreword to Dr. Saray Stancic's extraordinary book.

This is the era of lifestyle medicine: that is, using simple yet powerful lifestyle changes to reverse the progression of many of the most common chronic diseases as well as to help prevent these.

Lifestyle medicine is the most exciting movement today in health and healing—a revolutionary tidal wave that hasn't yet even begun to crest.

For more than four decades, I have directed a series of randomized controlled trials and demonstration projects proving, for the first time, that lifestyle medicine can often help prevent and even reverse the progression of the most common chronic diseases. It can be undertaken in combination with drugs and surgery, or sometimes as an alternative to these.

And the only side effects are good ones!

These lifestyle changes include:

- A whole foods, plant-based diet (naturally low in fat and refined carbohydrates)

- Stress management techniques (including meditation)

- Moderate exercise (such as walking)

- Social support and community (love and intimacy)

In short: eat well, stress less, move more, love more. That's it.

My colleagues and I continue to be amazed and inspired that the more diseases we study and the more underlying biological mechanisms we research, the more new reasons and scientific evidence we have to explain why these simple lifestyle changes are so powerful, how transformative and far-ranging their effects can be, and how quickly people can show significant and measurable improvements—often in just a few weeks or even less.

In our research, we use the latest high-tech, state-of-the-art scientific measures to prove the power of simple, low-cost and low-tech lifestyle interventions. Our studies have been published in the leading peer-reviewed medical and scientific journals and presented at the most well-respected physician conferences.

Our research is proving that many of the most common and debilitating chronic diseases and even much of the damages of aging at a cellular level may often be slowed, stopped, or possibly even reversed by this lifestyle medicine program. These include:

- Reversing even severe coronary heart disease

- Reversing type 2 diabetes

- Reversing early-stage prostate cancer

- Reversing high blood pressure

- Reversing elevated cholesterol levels

- Reversing obesity

- Reversing some types of early-stage dementia

- Reversing some autoimmune conditions, including arthritis

- Reversing emotional depression and anxiety

To this list we may now be able to add Dr. Saray Stancic's experience using lifestyle medicine to reverse the progression of multiple sclerosis. While this is an n of 1 study, not a randomized controlled trial, she shares in this book a powerful story of her healing journey.

Why is it that these same lifestyle changes may help prevent and even reverse the progression of such a wide range of chronic diseases?

Like most physicians, I was trained to view heart disease, diabetes, prostate cancer, and other chronic illnesses as being fundamentally different from each other. Different diagnoses, different diseases, different treatments.

But they're really not as different as they seem because they share many common origins and pathways.

We found that the same lifestyle changes described in this book can often reverse and thus help prevent the progression of a wide variety of the most common, costly, and disabling chronic diseases. Also, the more closely people adhered to this program, the more they improved in virtually every way we measured and the better they felt—at any age! These findings are giving many people new hope and new choices.

Why is this true?

The reason these same lifestyle changes are beneficial in so many chronic diseases is that they each affect and share so many common underlying biological causes, mechanisms, and pathways.

One of the important implications of this new unifying theory is to stop seeing chronic diseases as being fundamentally different from each other and to begin viewing them as diverse manifestations and expressions of similar underlying mechanisms, all of which are powerfully affected by the lifestyle choices we make every day—for better and for worse. (I describe this new unifying theory in more detail in our book, *UnDo It!*)

In other words, in many respects these are the same disease manifesting and masquerading in different forms. That is why the effects of lifestyle changes are not disease-specific—because they affect all of these mechanisms.

These biological mechanisms include changes in, among others:

- Chronic inflammation and immune system dysfunction

- Chronic emotional stress, depression, overstimulation of the sympathetic nervous system, stress hormones, and lack of sleep

- Gene expression and sirtuins

- Telomeres

- The microbiome

- Oxidative stress, cellular metabolism, and apoptosis

- Angiogenesis

- Stasis

Although this may seem like a radical theory, on further reflection it's not really that surprising. We know, for example, that regular exercise will help prevent and improve a wide variety of conditions—it's not disease-specific—whereas a sedentary lifestyle significantly increases the risk of many chronic diseases—also not disease-specific.

For the same reason, a whole foods, plant-based diet enhances our well-being in just about every aspect we can measure and helps prevent and even reverse the progression of so many different chronic diseases because this way of eating beneficially affects all of these mechanisms. Conversely, an unhealthy diet greatly increases the risk of a myriad of chronic illnesses via the same mechanisms.

Similarly, stress management techniques such as meditation and yoga improve our health in multiple ways, whereas sustained emotional stress significantly increases the risk of numerous chronic diseases via these same mechanisms.

Love and intimacy help keep us healthy, but people who are lonely and depressed are three to ten times likelier to get sick and die prematurely from virtually all causes.

Seeing from this perspective—that is, the same mechanisms affect a wide variety of chronic illnesses—also provides additional scientific evidence to explain why people often have several chronic diseases (called *comorbidities*) at the same time and why they share so many common risk factors. For example, many people with heart disease also have high blood pressure, type 2 diabetes, elevated cholesterol levels, obesity, and other chronic illnesses.

It also makes clear why these same lifestyle medicine changes may help prevent and improve all of these comorbidities simultaneously since they beneficially affect the same mechanisms which are underlying causes of these conditions. They all interrelate.

When I was in medical school learning how to do coronary bypass surgery, we were instructed in the standard procedure at that time: cut people open, bypass the clogged arteries in the heart, patch them up, and tell them they were cured. But over time, I noticed that many patients would return home after their surgery and eat the same junk foods, return to their sedentary lifestyle, not manage stress well, and soon enough, their bypasses often would clog back up.

When this happened, we'd often cut them open again and bypass the bypass, sometimes two or three times. So, for me, bypass surgery became a powerful metaphor for an incomplete approach. We were literally bypassing the problem without also treating the underlying causes: the lifestyle choices we make each day. And I began to wonder: Was there a better way? What would happen if we treated the causes?

In 1977, I began conducting a series of randomized controlled trials and demonstration projects showing that the progression of even severe coronary heart disease and other chronic diseases can often be reversed by making comprehensive lifestyle changes. I learned that our bodies often have a remarkable capacity to begin healing—and quickly—if we change the underlying lifestyle factors that cause a variety of chronic diseases.

Many years later, in 2013, I was speaking to over 1,500 people who were attending the annual conference of the American College of Lifestyle Medicine in Washington, DC. I respectfully appreciated that the conference directors referred to me as "the father of lifestyle medicine"—that is, using simple yet powerful lifestyle changes not only to help prevent but also to treat and often reverse the progression of the most common chronic diseases as well as to help prevent them.

After my presentation, a young woman came up to me and introduced herself. As we spoke, I got the distinct feeling that the woman before me, Dr. Saray Stancic, had found a home for her life's work.

As you will see in the pages that follow, Dr. Stancic is not only a practitioner of lifestyle medicine, she also began her journey as a patient. Stricken with a diagnosis of multiple sclerosis (MS) in 1995, she first tried the conventional methods of treatment. But as things got worse instead of better over the next few years, she took her treatment into her own hands and enacted the principles she now offers you in this book. By making significant changes to her lifestyle, Dr. Stancic now successfully manages her MS and is leading a healthy, active life, symptom-free and without pharmaceuticals.

What's particularly compelling about her story is that she did this on her own and didn't find out until later that there was already a small but committed group of lifestyle medicine doctors who were prescribing these interventions to our patients.

I've seen this joyful motivation in Dr. Stancic, because as I got to know her better over the next few years after our initial meeting, I admired how this passionate physician worked tirelessly to educate fellow health-care providers and her patients on the benefits of lifestyle medicine. Because she came to this approach through her own chronic illness, her perspective as both patient and physician provides invaluable insight into what it often takes to both heal from and prevent disease.

If you are ready to make changes in your life, Dr. Stancic is a wonderful guide. Your journey may start here if you apply the principles she teaches in this book.

—Dean Ornish, MD
Founder & President, Preventive Medicine Research Institute (nonprofit),
Clinical Professor of Medicine, University of California, San Francisco,
Author, *UnDo It!* and *The Spectrum*

www.ornish.com & www.pmri.org

Preface

Just after I submitted the manuscript for this book to my publisher in early 2020, the COVID-19 crisis spread across the globe.

As the former chief of infectious diseases at the VA Hudson Valley Health Care System in Montrose, New York, I am very familiar with pandemic preparedness. In my time there in the early 2000s, I worked closely on readiness and responsiveness during the anthrax and small-pox scares. And while the world community has experienced several close calls in recent decades with viruses like Ebola, SARS, and MERS, COVID-19 would make many of our worst fears a reality.

This event was also personal. I live in New Jersey, just outside New York City, and by April 2020 this area had become the epicenter of the outbreak in the United States. My husband, also a physician, had five staff members test positive within the span of a week. Health-care professionals, some of them close friends or coworkers, began succumbing to this plague at an alarming rate. I spoke on the phone with a patient in the hospital, whose words were muffled through an oxygen mask. "The guy in the room next door died last night, Dr. Stancic." It was heart-wrenching, and I felt helpless as I asked him to keep fighting, but reminded him of his wife and family awaiting his return.

COVID-19 hit my family directly. We lost our beloved Uncle Richard, a kind, giving soul who lived his entire life in Brooklyn. Not one anniversary, birthday, or Mother's Day had gone by without a card and thoughtful gift from a man who had little in the way of worldly possessions, but an abundance of love and compassion for his family. Sweet

Uncle Richard died alone on a stormy Monday morning in an ICU bed in Brooklyn. It haunted me that he and so many others were suffering and dying alone. They didn't have their loved ones beside them to ease their fears, no one to hold their hand, and no one able to say a proper goodbye. This is a great tragedy for patients and for their grieving families.

Then, in the face of this unfolding trauma, I began to notice something staggering. Preliminary studies of patients hospitalized with COVID-19 were indicating that the virus is not random or indiscriminate in whom it affects most severely. Demographic data from across the globe was revealing that the elderly and those living with existing diseases or chronic conditions are most likely to fare the worst when infected with the virus—particularly those with heart disease, chronic lung disease, hypertension (high blood pressure), obesity, and diabetes, all of which I diagnose regularly in new patients when they come to my practice.[1]

Of course, seeing people with these comorbidities is not unusual for most doctors, as more than 100 million Americans have high blood pressure, and obesity and diabetes rates climb each year, with no plateau in sight.[2] (A 2016 study in the *Lancet* showed that the United States is one of the most obese countries on the planet, and our numbers continue to rise.[3]) So this pandemic, while already tragic, had now taken on an even more devastating character. We are facing a novel, lethal, infectious disease that favors killing vulnerable populations in our society.

But here's the important difference between those living with chronic disease and the elderly: chronic conditions are in most cases the result of poor lifestyle choices. While many Americans have heard that poor choices such as eating an unhealthy diet and not exercising can lead to an early death, COVID-19 has shown us that "early" can mean "right now."

Please know that I understand talking about people's poor choices is a sensitive topic to tackle in the midst of universal loss and fear. But the truth is that we need to have a sobering and compassionate conversation on this subject now more than ever. A virus like this, unleashed in an environment where chronic diseases are commonplace, can wreak irreparable destruction. It doesn't have to be this way.

Yet, as I watched this tragedy unfold, it became clearer than ever that most people don't want to have the difficult conversations with their friends, family members, and even themselves that this crisis is demanding of us. This is also true for many of my fellow doctors, who often avoid having the harder conversations with their patients about their lifestyle choices and who fail to challenge their colleagues or medical establishments, such as hospitals, to do so either.

What do I mean by this? Here are a couple of examples.

The other day I watched an interview on a national news program with a COVID-19 patient in his early forties who had barely survived the ordeal and had been intubated in the process. He warned this could happen to anyone, as he was young and had no preexisting conditions. Yet it was also apparent from the video that he was obese, and despite this, the anchor never pressed the survivor to clarify that obesity is in fact a preexisting condition. Of course, if the anchor had done so, or even simply asked the man if he thought his excess weight might have contributed to his risk and difficult course, the public outrage would have been swift, and the anchor might have even lost her job.

In another example, a friend forwarded me a Facebook post that had gone viral, even making the national news. In the post, a man was pictured in a hospital gown and was warning others to take COVID-19 very seriously, as he had been at death's door. Yet when I clicked through the post to see his profile, the next photo on his timeline was of a huge double cheeseburger and fries. He'd captioned it with an explanation that since he was now feeling better, a friend had brought his favorite meal to the hospital. His immune system had just been through the wringer, and now he was eating a fatty fast-food meal, one of the worst things he could do for his body as it recovers. Does it surprise you that he was not discouraged from eating this, especially while still in the hospital? It doesn't surprise me. Sadly, I see this type of thing all the time.

Doctors don't like telling their patients that they need to lose weight (especially if the doctors themselves are overweight), and hospitals regularly either serve or allow meals for patients that contain the very ingredients that contributed to their hospitalization in the first place. Most doctors would rather write a prescription for prediabetes than counsel and support a real weight loss strategy, and this is part of a disturbing lack of perspective in medical education and practice. From solo physicians up to our largest hospitals, glaring omissions in education and treatment are literally killing us.

In my own practice, patients are often shocked when I tell them that they are obese and respond that no other doctor has ever told them this. I would rather tell someone the truth in the short term and help them stay alive and healthy than keep quiet and lose them to preventable death by staying "polite." I also know, however, that there is a disturbing trend in which obese people, faced with negative encounters and shaming experiences in a variety of health settings, may choose to avoid seeing a doctor at all, which only adds to the problem.[4] Personally, I have encountered a handful of obese patients who eat properly and engage in healthy lifestyle choices but still do not lose weight, and the reasons behind this are multifactorial and not clearly understood. So while I believe that this conversation is vital and necessary, I also absolutely believe that it is a conversation that should be engaged with kindness and understanding.

It shouldn't be controversial to say with firm and good-hearted conviction that we need to change, both as individuals and as a culture, especially in light of what we now know about COVID-19. We shouldn't have to live in a world where being normal weight puts you in a minority, or where a healthy blood pressure reading makes you remarkable, or where having type 2 diabetes is considered "nothing to worry about."

We need to bring paramount attention and resources to our minority communities deeply affected by a lack of access to healthy food and quality health care. On an individual level, we have to stop blaming our genes for our blood pressure, sugar level, and BMI, and take personal responsibility. On a societal level, we need to address the ways in which inequality, media messaging, and blind spots in medical practice contribute to the problem. Our current habits make us susceptible to chronic diseases and, yes, a prime target for a virus that seems intent on doing great harm.

By educating all people, whether medical professionals or patients, whether they have been diagnosed with a chronic illness or not, whether they're obese or not, of the profoundly impactful changes that can be made in our lives through the implementation of the lifestyle principles in this book, we can lift all of us into a much brighter future. This is good news. If we accept this shift in paradigm and enact the changes I outline here, we will have the chance to reclaim the health and well-being that is our birthright. In the midst of this catastrophe, I believe the teachings that follow have grown more important than ever before. If there is a silver lining to COVID-19's destructive path, my hope is that we can use this agonizing experience to spawn a healthier, more sustainable existence for ourselves and communities around the world.

Introduction

There is something missing from medicine.

More than at any time in history, we are suffering from illnesses such as heart disease, diabetes, obesity, autoimmune conditions, hypertension, and other chronic medical issues. Those of us who have received these diagnoses have tried a wide range of treatments: prescription drugs, supplements, intensive and costly therapies, and surgery, often with disappointing results and a lack of real improvement. In fact, sometimes we even get worse, and we end up taking more pills in order to treat the side effects of our treatments. When we read a story about another patient's miraculous recovery or a clinical trial that shows promise, we might get a glimmer of hope; but we're not sure what or whom to believe. It can feel overwhelming to try to absorb and understand the mountain of medical evidence about treatment of chronic diseases—mainstream and not—much of it conflicting. There just doesn't seem to be enough information we can trust, and our own doctors are often missing the information that can offer us any hope for a better long-term quality of life. No wonder so many of us end up feeling confused and helpless in the face of chronic illness.

It's this situation and the prevailing sense of overwhelming frustration surrounding it that ultimately led me to the questions that now guide my life and professional practice as a physician:

What if the most common medical treatments for chronic conditions are misguided in that they are only treating the symptoms of disease rather than identifying and fixing the underlying problem? Furthermore, what if the majority of the medical establishment is built on this very practice of treating symptoms rather than root causes?

Contemporary medicine has evolved into a system that relies almost entirely on pharmaceutical and surgical treatments. We see this in everything from how doctors are trained all the way through what insurance companies will and will not reimburse. For those of us suffering with chronic ailments, the treatment of symptoms and exclusion of causes can be devastating. Imagine going to the emergency room with a painful broken ankle, but instead of fixing the break the doctors offer you a more comfortable shoe to alleviate your pain.

Don't get me wrong: Modern medicine is extremely effective in many areas, especially when it comes to acute care. For instance, if your appendix ruptures, doctors can fix that. If you break an arm, you can go to your nearest emergency room and receive the help you need. These are simple examples, and modern medicine has also developed many complex therapies that save lives and improve quality of life every day for more people than ever before. However, when it comes to treating chronic illnesses such as heart disease, diabetes, autoimmune disorders, and the like, we have to face the fact that in these areas, something is clearly missing.

I know this because I have been practicing medicine for over twenty-five years. For the first decade, I viewed treatment through the same lens that most of my colleagues still do. I sought to treat symptoms rather than address the root causes that were making my patients sick. Of course, I wasn't doing this on purpose; I felt certain that I was helping people. It was only when I became suddenly diagnosed with multiple sclerosis at age twenty-eight that I realized how much is missing from our treatment of chronic illness.

My Story

My life changed forever on October 11, 1995.

In the middle of a busy hospital shift during my medical residency, I laid down for a brief nap during one of my breaks. When I awoke and tried to get up, an extraordinary thing happened. I couldn't feel my legs.

I remember looking down and seeing that my legs were in fact still there, but when I reached out to touch them all I felt was the dead weight of a stranger's limbs. I had no sensation in them at all. Instinctively, I lunged forward, but the moment my feet touched the floor, pain seared up from the ground as if I had stepped onto a bed of hot coals. I immediately pulled back, fear and panic rising through my body.

I called out for help and was rushed to the emergency room. Shortly after that, a tech wheeled me into the radiology suite for an urgent MRI of my brain and spinal cord. After two hours trapped in the machine, writhing in pain while being instructed to remain still, the MRI concluded and they wheeled me into the holding area.

Then I heard the radiologist yell excitedly, "Hurry, get the residents and medical students—this is a classic case of MS!"

That was how I learned I had multiple sclerosis.

Eager to educate his team of physicians-in-training, the radiologist had forgotten all about *me*—the patient—lying on a gurney a few feet away as he enthusiastically shared the diseased brain images. My brain. The diagnosis, coupled with the callous manner in which it was delivered, was a devastating blow.

My life would never be the same.

When I had walked through the hospital doors earlier that morning I was a vibrant, healthy, twenty-eight-year-old physician. Now I was a patient in the same hospital with a disabling, chronic disease for which there was no cure.

I was struck by the irony of switching roles from doctor to patient. I knew so much, but none of it helped me. All I could do was lie in bed wearing a flimsy hospital gown and feel very vulnerable. Over the next few days, dozens of doctors filed in and out to examine my "dead" legs and discuss my progress. They often talked about my case as if I were not even in the room. Just a few days earlier I had been one of those doctors: making my rounds, prodding and poking while discussing the patient's prognosis and therapeutic plan. As they worked, I thought of how my own patients felt as they faced similar terrifying moments. This new perspective was jarring—and more than a little enlightening.

The chief neurologist delivered the full extent of the bad news. Multiple sclerosis is a lifelong progressive disease, he told me, with a strong likelihood of degeneration and disability leading to the need for canes, crutches, wheelchairs, and ultimately long-term care. The future was bleak; but the "good news" was that the FDA had approved a new drug to slow the progression of the disease. He recommended I begin treatment immediately with daily injections that would continue for the rest of my life.

Being a doctor myself, I had no trouble trusting his recommendation without reservation.

He also warned that although the drug was effective, there was the potential for some serious side effects: fever, chills, muscle aches and pain, nausea, vomiting, diarrhea, anorexia, injection site reactions, hair loss, depression and suicidal thoughts, to name just a few. In my own training, I had memorized dozens of lists like this—but I had never truly experienced what they meant for my patients.

Nothing could have prepared me for the severity of these side effects.

I would inject the drug at 10 p.m., and by 2 a.m. I would wake with a combination of violent shaking, chills, and fever that continued through the night. Within two weeks, the side effects and lack of sleep were so debilitating that I decided I could not continue with the injections, and I picked up the phone to tell my neurologist that I was calling it quits. Before I could get a word in edgewise, he advised that quitting was not a prudent decision, reminding me of the wheelchair that awaited me. I had no good options. He offered a compromise: we could treat the side effects of this drug . . . with more drugs.

For the next several years, daily cocktails of prescription drugs took over my life.

By the time I was in my early thirties, I never left the house without a pillbox, dependent on nearly a dozen medications to get through a regular day. Even though this regimen was supposed to slow my MS, the disease steadily progressed. It wasn't long before I had grown dependent on a cane, walker, or crutches, and even the occasional diaper. I continued with my life and my career as best I could, but on the inside I began to lose hope. Faced with the prospect of getting sicker every day for the rest of my life, I fell deeper and deeper into darkness and despair.

Then, eight years later, a flicker of light arrived in the most unusual way.

Little Blueberries and Big Questions

One day, I came across a lesser known medical journal, one I would typically not take a second look at. It caught my attention that day, however, because the cover contained the words *multiple sclerosis* next to the word . . . *blueberries.* I remember thinking, *What in the world could MS have to do with blueberries?* I turned to the article with interest; the authors of the study had concluded there were benefits to MS patients who had been fed a diet rich in blueberries, and suggested the anti-inflammatory qualities of the blueberry may have had something to do with it. But I was disappointed to discover that the study was poorly designed. I was discouraged that anyone had spent time and money on such a ridiculous study, creating false hope for people like me in the process. I remember sharing a good, dismissive laugh with a colleague over lunch that afternoon about these findings.

As days went by, however, I couldn't get that blueberry study out of my mind. It wasn't that I thought that eating blueberries could cure my MS, but the study had provoked a much more important question. For the first time in my professional life, I wondered: *Is there a connection between diet and disease?*

You would think that if there were, I would know—after all, I was a dual board-certified physician (infectious diseases and internal medicine).

But I thought back, and during the ten years of my life dedicated to higher education in the field of medicine, I couldn't think of a single time that my professors had conveyed that message. Motivated by the desperation of my own condition, I decided to research the question myself.

I turned to the medical search engine and entered the words "multiple sclerosis" and "diet," and what came back astonished me. The first article I read was over fifty years old—by Dr. Roy Swank in the *New England Journal of Medicine* in 1952.[1] Swank had found that Norway had one of the highest rates of MS in the world at the time, but that it was mostly occurring in landlocked farming communities where people ate lots of meat, dairy, and saturated fat.[2] On the coast of Norway, however, where people were eating primarily fish and plants, Swank found a much lower incidence of MS, leading him to hypothesize that saturated fat was to blame.

Swank then took it one step further, testing his hypothesis by treating MS patients with a low-fat, plant-based diet over the next thirty-plus years. He published his findings in 1990, which showed that these patients lived longer and better, with *95 percent remaining mobile and physically active*.[3] These were patients with MS, a disease that the medical community had written off as progressive, debilitative, and incurable.

That statement, *95 percent remained physically active*, replayed in my mind over and over. Could this be true? Might dietary choices influence MS outcomes? This study sparked an insatiable desire to learn more. I scoured the peer-reviewed medical literature and found additional evidence with data from all over the world that animal fat intake was both a risk factor for getting MS and led to higher mortality rate for those with the disease. The reverse was true for those who consumed more vegetable protein and dietary fiber, meaning *plants!*[4]

The more I looked, the more I found a common thread: eating fewer animal products plus eating more plants equaled better MS outcomes. Yet here I sat, a licensed medical doctor and MS patient receiving some of the best care available in the world, and never once in my years of medical training, practice, or as a patient had I ever heard of this connection.

As I continued to immerse myself in the literature about MS, I began to understand that other variables such as weight, exercise, stress, substance use, and more influenced both risk and outcomes in MS in a very meaningful manner. Piece by piece, a larger puzzle was coming together to reveal a logical, evidence-based map to effective management for people suffering from MS. People like me.

One of the final pieces of this puzzle was genes. In medical school and as a patient, I learned that MS is hardwired in your genes, and therefore there is nothing you can do to prevent or reverse it. The science of epigenetics has challenged this notion, and researchers have shown that gene expression depends on outside variables. Simply put, this means that just because you have a genetic predisposition to an illness doesn't necessarily mean that it will be expressed. It's more accurate to say that genes are like a light switch; they can be turned on or off. This begs the question: What actions flip the switch for MS and other chronic disorders? Epigenetics underlines the key ways that things such as diet, exercise, and stress help activate certain genes. In other words, our daily choices are critically important in regards to healthy outcomes. To be clear, I'm not saying that genes don't play a role—certainly they do—but my experiences both personally and professionally have led me to conclude that the *choices we make* are what matter most!

Taken together, this new information gave me hope that my condition could improve. I knew that I had to try to create a healing regimen based on the things in my lifestyle over which I had control. I had to transform what I ate, how I exercised, and how I slept, as well as how I dealt with stress. I had to change my lifestyle in order to transform my life.

Turning Toward Hope

With what I had learned as my guide, I implemented a plan to improve my diet by reducing animal sources and processed food intake, replacing it with healthier plant-based choices. Next, I devised a beginner's exercise plan that I could safely accomplish at home. I addressed the areas of stress in my life and began a simple practice of daily meditation. And I educated myself on sleep hygiene and learned how to sleep without sleeping pills or other prescription medications.

I was committed to my plan, and worked on it a little every day. Slowly but steadily, an amazing thing occurred. I began to feel better.

At first it was something as subtle as being able to stay up past *Jeopardy*. On one particular morning I felt confident enough to leave the cane in the car. Then, two years into my lifestyle change came a special day I remember well. It was July 2, 2005, and I attended a wedding, where I did two things that may seem trivial to you but to me were extraordinary: *I wore heels* and *I danced with my husband*. These were things I had felt sure I would never do again. I grew more and more confident in the power of what I now know as "lifestyle medicine."

Over time, I tapered off every one of the medications on which I had once been dependent. My MS symptoms continued to recede.

Then one day I was caught off guard when my brother proposed that I should run a marathon. He had watched my metamorphosis from the beginning, and while he meant it as a means of positive encouragement, I was shocked that he would suggest such an irresponsible goal. I shot back, "Are you crazy?! I can't run a marathon—I have multiple sclerosis!"

In that flash of anger, I realized that even though I had come so far, I was still living my life first and foremost as "someone with MS." This label came with so many limitations, things I could do and things I couldn't. This needed to end; I would not allow this disease to define the course of my life. The exchange with my brother planted the seed, and although I didn't go out and buy running shoes the next day, I began to entertain the idea.

When I finally conjured the confidence to try to run, it didn't go well. My balance was off and I fell. The idea started to feel imprudent or impossible again, so I put it aside. I wondered if maybe I had gotten as far as I ever would with my lifestyle treatment. But as I stuck with my program and my MS continued to improve, I forgot about my running difficulties and tried again. Then again. There is a nature preserve down the street from my home, with a narrow path about one mile long encircling a small lake. I remember the first day I made it all the way around the path without falling or stopping—I felt invincible! I called my husband to inform him that I would someday run a marathon. I wasn't sure how, or when, but someday I would.

On May 2, 2010, about seven years after my blueberry aha moment, I crossed the finish line at the New Jersey Marathon. It was one of the most joyful days of my life—not because it had been any kind of lifelong goal to run a marathon, but because I had accomplished what seemed impossible just a few years earlier. My optimized lifestyle had been the crucial key to my recovery, and implementing these modifications has changed the trajectory of my life.

We Need a Revolution in Medicine

Today, these experiences fuel my desire to share this simple, yet powerful healing message with the world. Over more than two decades of practicing medicine, I have witnessed so much pain and suffering that I now know is preventable. What I have learned and will share with you in this book is for anyone affected by chronic disease—their own or that of a loved one. It's also for those of us who want to manage and take control of our risk factors for developing these kinds of diseases *before* they become debilitating. I am disappointed by a health-care system that functions more like a *sick*-care system, treating symptoms without focusing on underlying causes. This is the simple and powerful truth, and there is plenty of hard data to back it up: our lifestyle choices are a *critical component* in effective disease management and prevention. This is what's missing from medicine. The irony doesn't escape me that my own doctors—who were brilliant, well-trained, compassionate clinicians—were incapable of offering me the one therapeutic intervention that changed the course of my MS so profoundly.

What if all physicians everywhere joined together and spoke up for the clear and universal power of lifestyle medicine? This would be a miracle. It could be the catalyst for a sweeping shift in how we define true health care and could add what is missing so that our system can focus on preserving health, not only treating sickness. In order to turn the tide of chronic disease and the epidemic of illnesses such as obesity, autoimmune disorders, diabetes, and the stress that goes along with them, we must evolve. Doctors and patients alike need to embrace a paradigm shift. Right now we're passive and powerless—convinced that our genes define us, food choices don't really matter, and prescription drugs will save us. Truly, we can only take control of our personal health outcomes by optimizing all aspects of lifestyle. I choose the latter, and this book is your invitation to do so too.

If you are suffering from chronic illness and have been told by well-meaning health-care professionals that it's time to manage and "live with it," please know that I can relate. Whether you've been recently diagnosed or are many years into treatment, I believe the information in this book can help you. Likewise, if you know you are at high risk for certain chronic diseases because of your family history or other risk factors, this book is also for you. And if you are simply interested in a research-based medical approach for you and your family that incorporates more aspects of your well-being than just pill bottles and specialist visits, this book is for you as well.

In these pages, we will fill in the major holes in the current practice of medicine that leave too many of us suffering, disempowered, and even hopeless. It doesn't have to be like this. Here's the good news: most, if not all, of the needed changes are common sense. You don't have to go to medical school, memorize anatomy, or study surgical procedures. In fact, it's as if modern medicine, with all it has accomplished with complex procedures and advanced bioengineering, has overlooked the very basic practices to effectively treat and prevent chronic illness. In this book you will learn how to create and follow a plan for health and healing that not only addresses your disease but can also *transform your whole life*. I know this because I've seen it happen with my patients again and again. This was only after I did it for myself. You can do it too.

Using This Book

This book begins with a bit of scientific background about how chronic diseases have become so prevalent in industrialized societies like ours. As a doctor and patient, I know that almost none of us can make changes of any kind unless we understand the magnitude of the problem. After that, we'll get into specifics, with chapters dedicated to each of the six major areas of lifestyle change that have made all the difference for me and for my patients: optimizing nutrition, physical activity, stress management, and sleep hygiene; reducing or eliminating the intake of substances; and fostering social connections. You'll find stories and evidence of how each of these areas affects chronic illness and how making a few simple adjustments will result in profound, life-changing results. Most importantly, I've included tips, exercises, and easy-to-follow plans for making these changes. While it might feel overwhelming at first, I encourage you to do whatever you can at whatever pace you are able. Each day you work toward the goals in this book is a chance to move further away from the pain, suffering, and isolation of chronic disease. You deserve that.

My wish for you, and for each and every one of us, is the same: may we live joyful, productive lives free of chronic disease. May we eat well, relish physical and mental challenges, enjoy restorative sleep, and connect deeply with others. Then, maybe at the age of ninety-five or older, after a glorious day spent with family and friends, we can pass away peacefully in our sleep. That sounds like the perfect end to a well-lived life.

The Man-Made Epidemic of Chronic Disease

Awareness is the greatest agent for change.
—Eckhart Tolle

This is a book about hope, empowerment, and transformation.

Too many of us have been suffering for too long from diseases, conditions, and ailments that we have been told are progressive, incurable, and unavoidably genetic. We have resigned ourselves to a diminished life and closed ourselves off to what we believe is possible for us to experience or achieve. We have come to define ourselves by our symptoms, rather than by our potential.

It's time to change our future, and the principles in this book are a guide to doing exactly that.

I have used the methods that follow to manage my own diagnosis of multiple sclerosis, a disease that kept me reliant on a cane and a cocktail of prescription drugs for years. Today, I am happy to say, I exercise regularly and take no medications for my MS. I have dedicated my professional life and medical practice to helping others implement these same lifestyle changes and beat chronic illness.

However, in order to do what I and so many of my patients have done, you need to understand what you're up against. One thing I encounter again and again is the difficulty on the part of some patients to make and sustain changes they know are good for them. Of course, our choices are our own individual responsibility, but every choice we make also takes place in the wider social context in which we live. For example, the decline in rates of smoking over the last several decades is due not only to individuals making the choice to quit, but also to larger societal shifts in culture and public policy, such as warning labels, education on the danger of smoking, and restricting areas where smoking is allowed. When it comes to the prevalence and treatment of chronic illness, we need to take a good hard look at our current medical system, as well as the many ways the food and pharmaceutical industries intersect with people's daily choices, for better or for worse. Without understanding this wider context, it can be difficult to sustain the motivation you need for long-term individual change.

In other words, in order for you to be fully willing and able to enact these principles in your own life, you must know and understand how we arrived at the current situation. When we are suffering with a chronic disease, the idea of starting and maintaining something new—even if we know it will probably be good for us and make us feel better—can be daunting. Fortunately, simply changing your perspective on health and healing, and understanding what's going on in the bigger picture, can alleviate the sense of being overwhelmed.

Communicable versus Noncommunicable Diseases

For most of human history, when people got sick and died, they did so from infectious diseases that were largely passed along through the population (others died from minor injuries, which could easily be fatal without antibiotics and the other kinds of straightforward treatments we have today). At the beginning of the twentieth century, the top three causes of death in the United States were pneumonia/influenza, tuberculosis, and diarrhea (a common symptom of the dreaded "stomach bug" most of us have contracted at least once in our lives).[1]

RANK	TOP TEN CAUSES OF DEATH IN THE U.S. (1900)
1	Pneumonia and Influenza
2	Tuberculosis
3	Diarrhea
4	Heart Disease
5	Intracranial Lesions of Vascular Origin (Stroke)
6	Nephritis (Kidney Disease)
7	Accidents
8	Cancer
9	Senility
10	Diptheria

Over the course of that century, we developed revolutionary remedies to communicable diseases, like antibiotics that effectively treated these ailments, thereby increasing our expected life span and improving our quality of life. Minimizing the impact of these communicable diseases is perhaps the greatest accomplishment of modern medicine.

Fast-forward to the twenty-first century, and the picture changes. To a greater extent than you may realize, we are living in a time that can best be defined as the era of a man-made epidemic of chronic disease. You probably know that a chronic disease refers to any condition that is expected to last for a long time, even the rest of someone's life. Until the twentieth century, infectious diseases such as polio were included in this umbrella. So a better term to define the modern state of affairs would be noncommunicable diseases (NCDs).[2] Unlike the communicable diseases of the past, which were mostly transmitted from person to person via an infectious agent, today's chronic disease epidemic is predominantly a man-made, self-inflicted phenomenon. These NCDs are largely due to the fact that we choose to engage in behaviors and habits that are literally killing us. We're not getting sick from germs or infected wounds; we're partaking in risky behaviors such as poor nutrition, lack of exercise, social isolation, poor sleep hygiene, high stress, and ingesting harmful substances.

RANK	TOP TEN CAUSES OF DEATH IN THE U.S. (2017)	NUMBER OF DEATHS
1	Heart Disease	647,457
2	Cancer	599,108
3	Accidents	169,936
4	Chronic Lower Respiratory Diseases	160,201
5	Stroke	146,383
6	Alzheimer's Disease	121,404
7	Diabetes	83,564
8	Influenza and Pneumonia	55,672
9	Nephritis, Nephrotic Syndrome (Kidney Disease)	50,633
10	Intentional Harm (Suicide)	47,173

Take a look at the CDC's top ten causes of death in the United States as of 2017, which shows that heart disease and cancer were the number one and two leading causes of death, accounting for nearly 50 percent of all deaths.[3]

Even when we account for the fact that advances in medicine have greatly reduced or eliminated the spread and mortality of infectious diseases, we still see an incredibly disproportionate rise in heart disease, obesity, diabetes, and autoimmune diseases. These are largely diseases of excess, often the result of too much sugar, too much salt, too much fat, too much sitting, and too much stressing. In a way, the tendency toward these behaviors makes sense from an evolutionary standpoint. For tens of thousands of years, humans had little access to foods with high fat, sugar, or salt content. Every calorie counted, and sitting down meant saving energy. Our brain evolved triggers to load up on ripe fruits or fatty nuts whenever we found them. Today, surrounded by foods that stimulate these triggers but have none of the nutritional value of fruits or nuts, our brains and bodies run into real trouble. We see the consequences of this in the CDC's current list of lifestyle- and behavior-related top killers. Almost half of Americans have high blood pressure, high cholesterol, or addiction to cigarettes—the leading risk factors for heart disease.[4] All of these risks can be significantly reduced with lifestyle changes.

We know what is killing us, and we know how to prevent it. Yet, we choose to continue down this catastrophic path to a predictable dead end. This is a kind of madness.

The Worsening Crisis

Beyond heart disease and cancer, our lifestyle choices have also been strongly linked to stroke, Alzheimer's disease, and diabetes. Diabetes in particular is growing at an alarming rate. In the early nineties, fewer than 3 percent of the population in the United States had diabetes.[5] Today, we are brushing past 10 percent, and the CDC ominously predicts that by 2050 more than 30 percent of Americans will be living with diabetes.[6] That's more than 100 million Americans. Apart from the physical toll on patients themselves, this current trend is unsustainable for society and the health-care system, as diabetes care is among the most expensive chronic diseases, fueling huge increases in health-care costs. Remarkably, annual health-care costs in the United States have now surpassed the $3 trillion mark, with approximately 90 percent of those dollars allocated to chronic disease management.[7] To understand these costs and the complications of diabetes, let's look at a common scenario. As an infectious disease specialist, I often saw patients with a nonhealing infected foot ulcer. This is a common complication of diabetes that can infect the bone and result in amputation of a toe, foot, or even leg. At this point in the disease, patients face huge obstacles to reversing course and an avalanche of poor health outcomes including blindness, renal failure, heart attack, stroke, and death. We know that diabetes is 93 percent preventable, so scenarios like these should be rare, and yet they happen every day in every hospital across the country and no one bats an eye.[8] Furthermore, no diabetic starts out facing an amputation or stroke. There are years if not decades to intervene and mitigate the risk factors of poor food choice, sitting, and stress.

It appears our growing waistlines are a large contributor to our current crises. Medicine has long known that extra weight contributes to a number of health issues and is a risk factor for many of the CDC's top killers. In chapter 3, we'll take a more detailed look at how and what we eat affects health outcomes and what we can do about it. For now, it's important to note that the spike in noncommunicable diseases correlates with an alarming rise in obesity over the last thirty years.

Sometime in the early eighties, doctors and public health officials reached a consensus about trends in harmful health behaviors and their role in premature death. In 1984, as a response to this understanding, a CDC program interviewed people by phone to assess the role behaviors might have on health outcomes.[9] The obesity trends this program revealed tell an alarming story: In 1990, no state had obesity rates greater than 15 percent. By 2010, no state had obesity rates less than 20 percent.

Most recent data report 22 states now have obesity rates between 30 and 35 percent. Believe it or not, nine states have the menacing distinction of obesity rates greater than 35 percent (Alabama, Arkansas, Iowa, Louisiana, Mississippi, Missouri, North Dakota, Kentucky, and West Virginia).[10] Remarkably, the most recent obesity rate for the United States is 42.4 percent![11] If we combine Americans who are overweight with those who are obese, we surpass more than 70 percent of the population.[12]

That means if you are a healthy weight in the United States, you are in the minority. Allow that to sink in. Fewer than half the people in our country can enjoy the basic benefits of health and well-being that come from sustaining an ideal body weight.

The CDC reports 60 percent of Americans are living with at least one chronic disease, and 40 percent with at least two.[13] That means more than half of our population is sick. Does that make any sense? This is nothing short of a medical, economic, and societal disaster. How can we hope to keep up with such vast rates of illness? Will we have enough doctors? Will it bankrupt us? Doctors, hospitals, and insurance companies are frantically trying to mop up this crisis, all while failing to see or address its cause.

Autoimmune Diseases

Another looming concern is the recent dramatic increase in autoimmune diseases such as type 1 diabetes, MS, lupus, rheumatoid arthritis, and Graves' disease. A systematic review of thirty studies published in 2015 revealed a significant increase of these over the last thirty years, and researchers blame environmental factors, in particular our lifestyle choices, as part of the cause.[14] I'd like to say a word here about genetics, as they are often mentioned in discussions of autoimmune diseases and their causes. While genes can predispose a person to developing an illness such as an autoimmune disease, they are by no means a guarantee. We know this because of studies of identical twins who share the exact same DNA. If only genes were at play, twin A would almost always have the same autoimmune disease as twin B. There are some exceptions, but in general identical twin studies report only around a 20 to 30 percent chance of both twins having the same autoimmune disease.[15] So it's not just our genes! Without heaping blame or shame on patients suffering from these issues, we can nonetheless acknowledge that we each have a part to play in changing our behaviors and optimizing our environment. Hopefully you can take this as an empowering finding; we are not totally beholden to our genes.

When it comes to autoimmune disease in Western industrialized societies, there are three leading theories about why we are seeing a steep rise: hygiene, psychosocial stress, and obesity.[16] In short, researchers are suggesting that we are perhaps too sterile, too stressed, and too heavy.

The hygiene hypothesis is interesting. In general, in industrialized countries we have improved hygienic conditions and access to vaccines and antibiotics, so there are lower rates of infections. However, fewer exposures to organisms or pathogens like bacteria and viruses may lead to an immature or faulty immune system. Maybe we *need* to experience these infections in order to develop a healthy, robust immune system. I regrettably recall almost losing my mind when my two-year-old son licked the grocery cart handle at the supermarket. What if he were only strengthening his immune response, and I just didn't know it? Nowadays we routinely cover our children and everything in their environment with sanitizer or bleach wipes. This may be part of the problem.

The psychosocial theory proposes that our fast-paced, stressful world may be a culprit in fueling the autoimmune epidemic. This hypothesis was tested in a recent study looking at MS patients and stress. The trial randomized half the patients to receive stress management therapy while the other half received none. After twenty-four weeks they compared MRI findings from the beginning and the end of treatment. They found three-quarters of the patients who received the therapy had no evidence of progression (no new lesions) of MS in their brain, while in the control group only half had no evidence of disease progression. The significant conclusion of this study suggests that stress management really does matter.[17]

It's worth noting that, as with our genes, we can't always control the amount or kinds of stress we encounter; but we do have a choice in how we respond to stress and the ways in which we manage it through approaches like meditation, therapy, or other behavioral changes. We will cover many of these techniques in chapter 5.

Finally, our third leading theory is *obesity*. We have already talked about the indisputable role of extra weight in fueling diseases like heart disease and diabetes, but researchers are now recognizing this excess fat may be contributing to autoimmunity issues as well.[18] While we don't fully understand why, the bottom line is that autoimmune diseases are exploding, affecting 50 million Americans and costing the nation $100 billion per year. By way of perspective, cancer affects 9 million Americans and costs the country $57 billion in health-care costs. Seeing these numbers, it will be no surprise to learn the top-selling pharmaceutical drug in the United States is Humira, an immunosuppressive medication used to treat several autoimmune diseases.[19] Global sales for this drug alone were reported at an astonishing $18.43 billion in 2017. These diseases are not only compromising our health and quality of life, they are also emptying our bank accounts and restructuring the economic foundation of our health-care systems. We will be returning to autoimmune diseases throughout this book, because I know that many of you are suffering from one or more.

Cancer

Before we move further, we need to take a moment to talk about cancer, as this is the second leading cause of death in the country. The risks of developing two of the most common cancers—breast and colon—have been shown to be significantly reduced by exercise. Other cancers can be mitigated through lifestyle changes as well, including optimal nutrition that avoids animal products, especially red meat and dairy, stress reduction, cessation of alcohol consumption and smoking, and even good sleep hygiene.

Lifestyle is of primary importance in reducing your risk of getting cancer, but we also understand its value in reducing recurrence and increasing survival for women living with breast cancer. The Women's Healthy Eating and Living (WHEL) Study showed optimizing lifestyle after a breast cancer diagnosis reduced mortality by as much as 50 percent.[20] Positive outcomes in prostate cancer prevention and treatment are also closely tied to healthy lifestyle choices. I believe that if you are battling cancer now, making the changes outlined in this book can help you. That being said, I want to stress how important it is that you be open with your practitioners about any lifestyle changes you are making while in their care. What I want you to remember as we go forward is this: there is strong evidence that basic healthy habits contribute to a reduced risk of cancer over the span of life and to better outcomes after treatment.

The Profit Factor in Medicine and How We Educate Doctors

While I genuinely believe that most doctors are *not* in the field for the money, any discussion about the problem in medicine would be incomplete without a look at the financial incentives built in for surgery and pharmaceuticals. Sadly, I feel that the main reason nutrition and preventive measures are rarely, if ever, practiced is because there are no financial incentives to do so. In fact, time spent practicing preventive medicine takes away from billable hours, which ends up as a financial deterrent to stopping chronic illness before it starts.

For instance, did you know that bypass surgery brings in an average of $150,000 per operation?[21] Perhaps more than any other, this procedure keeps hospitals in the black. When you take this into consideration, it's no wonder some doctors and health systems wear blinders when it comes to lifestyle choices and their effects on human health.

In an interview with the *Washington Post*, my dear friend and prominent lifestyle medicine advocate Dr. Dean Ornish offered a fitting metaphor for our Western medical system: we're "bypassing" the real problems when we focus on surgery and prescription drugs as treatment, rather than acknowledging the underlying causes of disease. A simple shift in approach could revolutionize clinical medicine from being a reactive discipline to a proactive, preventive one. Empowering an educated patient to take control of their personal health outcomes is the key, and this includes making sure our doctors are educated too.

In my own medical training, I had never even heard of the long-established links between diet and MS, let alone how nutrition might affect other diseases. When you consider this gap in our education, it's no wonder that so many of our own health-care facilities have horrible food environments. Well over half of medical schools maintain a fast-food franchise in one of their affiliated hospitals. For years, the prestigious Cleveland Clinic housed a McDonald's, and it wasn't until 2015 and after much debate that it was removed.[22] At my alma mater, Rutgers New Jersey Medical School, there is still a Burger King in the hospital's cafeteria, despite a recent protest and a petition signed by more than three thousand people requesting its removal. At lunchtime, a line of white coats can easily order Whoppers and deep-fried onion rings. If you're old enough, you may remember that doctors used to smoke in hospitals too. Hard to believe, right? The supersized order of fries is the modern-day cigarette, and we have yet to fully acknowledge it so that we can correct course.

Regrettably, only about one-fourth of medical schools offer the recommended twenty-five total hours of nutrition education over four years of study.[23] This is shocking in light of the numerous studies showing how dietary interventions have served to both prevent and improve outcomes in chronic disease. For example, if you have a heart attack, you can reduce your risk of a second heart attack by 72 percent if you just improve your diet.[24] *That's a far better outcome than any drug on the market.* Given the effectiveness of dietary changes to reduce heart attacks, one would think that cardiologists should be well versed in the field of nutrition; but doctors can actually complete a graduate cardiology specialty without ever studying nutrition at all. Further, to become a full-fledged cardiologist, you must complete one hundred invasive cardiac catheterization procedures, but zero hours of nutrition.

Here, again, what goes for heart disease also goes for diabetes and other chronic illnesses. A well-known study concluded that a dietary and physical activity intervention was nearly twice as effective as a pharmaceutical drug in preventing diabetes in individuals at risk.[25] Yet most doctors just write for the drug, despite having a randomized clinical trial that says diet and exercise are better for patients!

This brings me to an important point. Not only do hospitals profit from costly surgeries and landlord/tenant relationships with the fast-food industry, but our health-care system also relies on an ethically problematic exchange with drug companies to the tune of billions of dollars per year.[26] For example, pharmaceutical companies often offer incentives to doctors they classify as a "promotion" of their products.[27] From free staff lunches to elaborate meals in expensive restaurants and generous speaking fees as direct payment to doctors who include promotion of their drugs to other health-care professionals, big pharma has invested huge amounts of money in marketing their drugs directly to physicians, which is effectively compensating them for writing those prescriptions. While the establishment of reporting websites like Open Payments (a national transparency program provided by the Centers for Medicare & Medicaid Services) have led to some changes, 48 percent of doctors in the United States still received a total of $2.4 billion from the pharmaceutical industry alone in 2015.[28] Sadly, there is little doubt that these incentives are impacting a doctor's decision to write certain prescriptions.[29]

A question with which I have long struggled is how the importance of making healthy lifestyle choices competes with this kind of influence on the priorities of doctors and hospitals. As my friend Dr. Michael Greger notably pointed out to me, "When's the last time, your doctor was taken out to dinner by big broccoli? It's probably been a while." That is a larger question our society needs to answer. But in the meantime, there is something you can do to take control of your own health, and this book will help you do exactly that.

Knowledge Is Power

Reading this gloom and doom account of the health-care dilemma we face today might make you want to throw up your hands, especially if you're living with a chronic disease yourself. My intention, however, is to give you an objective, comprehensive view of the problem because I believe that *knowledge is power*. I also know that people are often inspired to change from a place of desperation, as I was. The state of the world and your own health can fuel your own powerful personal transformation. Although the situation appears grim, the solution is very accessible. We know exactly what we need to do to change the lives of millions of people across the world. For your own sake, I also want you to know that while these problems are systemic and pervasive, *you are not alone.* There is a way forward.

My other hope with this book is to show you that not only is the solution available to you right now, but it can also be *enjoyable*. Taking care of your health doesn't have to be the heavy, expensive, exhausting burden it's often made out to be in our culture. It can be joyful, rewarding, delicious, and fun! Healthy nutrition can be a wealth of colors, textures, and tastes. Movement can be play. Stress can be transformed into peace. I know this with 100 percent certainty because I've seen it in my own life as well as those of my patients.

This book will teach you the six main areas of lifestyle medicine and how you can implement them in your life. And here's the exciting thing about this approach: it applies to basically all chronic diseases. Doctors are trained in medical school that each area of medicine is separate. The benefit of specialization is that we have ultraprecise tools and practices at our disposal, which we certainly need. We memorize long lists of drugs and learn procedures to treat heart problems that don't cross over into treatment of cancer or diabetes. This seems to make sense on the surface, but the research into lifestyle medicine shows that there is a much better way. The improvements gained by changes in lifestyle factors are felt in the whole body. If you are using lifestyle medicine to manage MS, for example, your risk for developing heart disease or diabetes also drops significantly. That's the simplicity and beauty of this approach to health and healing.

It's time to retake control of our illnesses, our health, and our lives—individually and as a society. Together we can do this. Our society needs a wake-up call. The lifestyle changes I will recommend are not only common sense but are supported by an overwhelming body of evidence in the peer-reviewed medical literature. It's time for my peers to pull their heads out of the sand and start extolling the virtues of optimal lifestyle choices. It's time to redefine the medical education model so that we equip doctors and health-care professionals with the knowledge they need to combat the man-made epidemic of chronic illness.

Are you with me?

The Lifestyle Medicine Solution

You must do the thing you think you cannot do.
—Eleanor Roosevelt

When I lecture to medical students about the benefits of lifestyle medicine, I often include a slide of the Hippocratic oath. Doctors all over the world have the great honor of reciting this sacred promise at the time of their graduation. While the modern version spans 341 words, none are more important to me than these:

> *I will prevent disease whenever I can,*
> *for prevention is preferable to cure.*

We can all understand the simple truth that it's better not to get sick at all than to suffer and be cured. Indeed, if doctors aim to nurture the health and well-being of our patients, prevention ought to trump all else in health care.

When I was in medical school, I took a course called Preventive Medicine, but I soon learned we were really talking about *secondary prevention*, also known as early detection. For example, my professor lectured on the importance of colonoscopy to "prevent" colon cancer. But colonoscopies don't prevent cancer; they detect it early. The same can be said for mammograms, digital prostate exams, and more. Certainly, these tests are valuable, but wouldn't it be far better to avert cancer altogether? That's what we call *primary prevention*. Not only is primary prevention barely covered during our years in training, it is effectively discouraged by the conflicting motives that are present in daily medical practice. Real prevention of course means halting the development of a chronic disease before it starts.

As you know by now, I believe there is a much more effective solution for prevention of chronic illnesses, and lifestyle medicine is that solution. In my own case, I was able to apply this solution and reverse the chronic illness that I had lived with for eight agonizing years.

This approach to health and healing restores what is missing from medicine by incorporating simple behaviors around how we eat, move, sleep, and take care of ourselves mentally and emotionally, all in an effort to achieve optimal health. It brings real, tangible hope back into the lives of those who are suffering. I know these protocols can prevent and even slow or reverse chronic illness because I have lived them and seen countless patients do so as well. The lifestyle medicine practices in this book can and will transform your life, and on a wider scale they have the potential to reverse the doomsday picture of health in our world.

The term *lifestyle medicine* may be new to you, so let's get you acquainted. Lifestyle medicine is an evidence-based, clinical discipline that supports the adoption of healthy lifestyle behaviors to prevent, treat, and reverse chronic diseases and improve quality of life. It is not in opposition or contrary to mainstream medicine. In my view, lifestyle medicine is what is missing in clinical medicine, and I absolutely believe that combining mainstream medical practices with lifestyle medicine has the potential to usher in a new era of sustainable health-care systems, revolutionize how we deal with chronic illness, and redefine our cultural view of health in general. Imagine the power of a system in which the medical miracles of vaccinations, surgeries, and specialized interventions could be combined with broad support for preventive and life-saving healthy habits that boosted the health and well-being of millions.

The Lifestyle Medicine Wheel

The lifestyle medicine approach includes six areas of importance. I like to think of these six topics as spokes on the lifestyle medicine wheel. They include a healthy diet, regular physical activity, stress management, good sleep hygiene, minimizing substance intake, and maximizing social connections. Just as with an actual wheel, each spoke forms an essential part of the functioning whole. When one spoke breaks down, the ride gets bumpy pretty fast. Although many patients start this process by focusing on food, as I did with my blueberry aha moment, the greatest benefits are achieved when we tend to each spoke simultaneously and in balance.

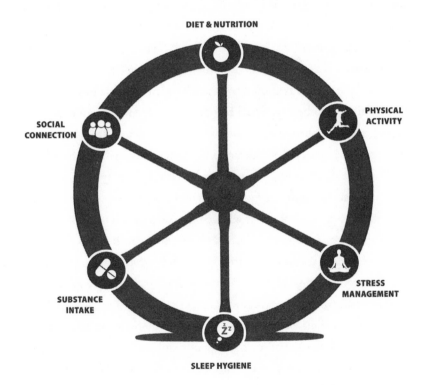

The goal of lifestyle medicine is to live your optimal existence, free of chronic disease and unnecessary pain and suffering. The first two spokes, diet and nutrition and physical activity, are the ones you have certainly heard before in the context of your health, but lifestyle medicine has some additional unique contributions that we'll cover. The other four spokes of the wheel—stress management, sleep hygiene, substance intake, and social connection—are not areas that come to mind for most people when it comes to their physical health. But as you will see in the chapters that follow, they are just as important to your overall health as the first two. For now, let's take a brief look at each spoke on our wheel.

Diet and Nutrition

Nutrition is the piece that gets the most press. In general, it's one of the most loaded topics we deal with in our society today. It makes me profoundly sad that what should be the simplest, most elemental basis for good health, prevention, cure, and longevity has been hijacked in every possible way. There are hundreds of diets, protocols, programs, and solutions out there—many touted by celebrities and notable physicians and most claiming to be supported by scientific evidence. Beyond the messaging from the outside world, we get plenty of advice from our family, friends, and inner circles. Everyone feels they know what is best for us and has a powerful anecdote or diet guru to back it up. We all come from different backgrounds, and as a result nothing feels more fraught and complicated than figuring out what comprises a healthy diet.

Patients often ask me questions like: How can it be that so many diet recommendations often directly contradict one another? How can the science be saying *eat more dairy* and *don't eat any dairy* at the same time? My answer to these questions is that people often cherry-pick data that supports their beliefs, especially when there are financial incentives for doing so. One of my guiding principles when evaluating claims about nutrition is to follow the money. If an individual or organization financially benefits from a dogmatic approach to food, it should give you pause when listening to their message.

To be clear, I have no horse in this race. I don't sell any type of food or supplements, nor do I receive any compensation from any of these groups. I believe in presenting the best research available on nutrition and empowering people to make informed decisions for themselves. In this book, I aim to convey objective, simple truths and hopefully answer many of your questions so that you can be confident that what is on your plate is serving to reduce your risk of disease and improve your overall well-being. I will also share my personal experience with how changing my diet helped me overcome MS and why I believe this can work for other chronic illnesses too.

Much of the work we have to do as we begin a lifestyle transformation involves shifting our perspective. Many of us, especially women, have grown up in a pernicious diet culture. Even well-meaning cultural icons have contributed to a distorted view of food and health. The saturation of media in our lives has made food and body image messaging impossible to ignore. Add to this the troubling rise in obesity and its very real associated risks, and we are understandably obsessed with the number on the scale. We resort to deprivation and starvation to try to control calories and attain impossible ideals, which often ends up backfiring into a yo-yoing state of endless losses and gains.

The number on the scale can no longer be what we pursue to the exclusion of our health. The question needs to change from "How many calories should I stay under each day so I can lose ten or twenty pounds?" to "What should I eat to live a long, healthy, and joyful life?" We can then embrace food again and consume the bountiful amounts needed to fulfill and satiate our needs, all while maintaining a healthy weight and reducing our risk of chronic disease. We reap enormous benefits when we shift our goal from hitting a number on the scale to overall wellness. What's more, when we engage that shift and choose foods that support wellness, increase our energy level, and make us feel better, weight loss is very often the pleasurable side effect of this process.

So there is plenty of complexity to the question of food in our society. And yet, I am here to stand up and say: Healthy eating is actually very simple. In fact, my prescription for a healthy diet can be summed up in just three words: *Eat mostly plants.*

Of course, with so much misinformation, you might have your doubts about this advice—and given all the mixed messages in our society about nutrition, I can understand why. For now, all I ask is that you join me in the conversation with an open mind. In the next chapter, we'll take a look at exactly how my simple three-word prescription, "eat mostly plants," works in real life. But first, let's continue with a look at the other five spokes of our lifestyle medicine wheel.

Physical Activity

Regular physical activity helps maintain a healthy weight and strong body, and there's a lot of research that there are myriad other benefits as well, including improved mood, increased energy, sharpened attentiveness, and better sleep, to name a few. In the longer term, regular physical activity can also reduce your risk of heart disease, diabetes, stroke, dementia and Alzheimer's, as well as many cancers, including two of the most common worldwide—breast cancer and colon cancer.[1] More importantly, moving is fun and can even be addictive in a good way, which helps make it a self-sustaining practice.

Despite exercise's well-documented benefits, only 23 percent of Americans meet these minimum recommendations: 150 minutes of moderate intensity physical activity per week, as well as muscle strengthening or resistance activities twice a week.[2] It should come as no surprise that a report listing best exercise practices for all fifty states correlates closely with the CDC's obesity map. Colorado has the lowest obesity rate and the highest percentage of adults meeting the physical activity guidelines, at 32.5 percent. Conversely, the least active state, Mississippi, with only 13.5 percent of adults meeting movement guidelines, claims one of the highest obesity rates. Inactivity and obesity go hand in hand.

In terms of your personal transformation, even small changes in your level of activity can make a big difference. Something as simple as parking the car a bit farther from the storefront, or taking the stairs instead of the elevator, is a literal step in the right direction. Consistency is key. Doing even a few minutes of extra movement each day will yield better health outcomes than a rigorous exercise routine that you stop after a couple weeks. Part of the trick is to make lasting changes that you can incorporate into your everyday routine.

Play > Exercise

A pediatrician I know purposely avoids using the word *exercise* with kids; instead, he talks about *play*. Exercise can seem like more work than fun, and shifting the focus to an activity of leisure or joy can help kids and adults alike. With my patients, I often start out by asking them what they do for fun, or what their favorite activity was when they were a kid, and why. If you enjoyed riding your bike with friends or playing catch with your dad in the backyard, this might be a great time to rekindle that feeling. Dust off that vintage bicycle and head to the local bike path on a beautiful sunny afternoon. A dear friend of mine started playing tennis at forty-three, and now at fifty he's in better shape than he was seven years earlier. You're never too old to start a fun movement routine, and the key is often to find a way to incorporate play into the equation.

In my own case, I love to hike but never thought I'd be able to again after my MS diagnosis. Physical activity was scary to me, with the real threat of falling and injury. When I was first diagnosed, it was thought that MS patients should not exercise because it could make the disease worse. So for eight years I tried *not* to move very much. This left me weak and demoralized. When I created my first treatment plan, I got a stationary bike. My husband had to help me get on it, and after one minute those first days I had to get off, in pain and exhausted. It took ten to fifteen minutes to recover. The next day, he would help me on again. Day after day, I slowly built up my stamina and strength.

Even in cases of advanced disability and chronic illness, there are almost always ways that you can ease into moving and challenging yourself. Everything from stretching or yoga in a chair to working with modified exercise equipment can be your ally here. So if you cringe at the thought of exercise or physical activity, remember these two things:

small and consistent changes matter, and find a way to play! We'll dive into this topic more fully in chapter 4.

Stress Management

Stress is an invisible monster that lurks in the shadows. We can't see it, touch it, or measure it like we can our temperature, so this makes it that much harder to spot and rein in. Even when we are aware of stress, we very often try to ignore it or push through it, as many of our societal and cultural messages encourage exactly this form of self-flagellation. The argument seems to be that stress is all mental. Let me explain why this thinking is just plain wrong.

When you have a stressful thought, it doesn't just sit above you in a cloud like a cartoon bubble, but instead triggers a cascade of biological events that lead to the fight-or-flight response in your body. Your brain releases chemical signals that travel throughout the body, triggering the production of the stress hormones epinephrine (adrenaline) and cortisol. Your blood pressure and heart rate go up, and your palms get sweaty. Cortisol stimulates the release of stored blood sugar from your liver, and the pancreas kicks in to even things back out by producing insulin. Over time, increased levels of these hormones lead to cellular damage and inflammation, which fuel chronic diseases.

Evolutionarily speaking, this type of fight-or-flight response makes a lot of sense, as it supported our survival. If a saber-toothed tiger appeared to ancient humans, the ability to perceive this threat and respond quickly meant staying alive. But in today's world, our body makes no distinction between true life-threatening situations and everyday stressors as varied as traffic, looming deadlines at work, or the aggravating comment on your Facebook post. All of these events can trigger a similar biological response.

The Stress Solution

This book will offer you some solutions to reduce the stress in your life by using two main approaches: learning to change what you can and developing practices of mindfulness and meditation. When I first introduced a lifestyle treatment plan for myself, I had to change what I could around the factors that were causing stress in my life. This meant telling my colleagues at the hospital that I would be going home at 5 p.m. each day (barring a patient emergency) and that I would be declining any opportunities to add additional research projects to my workload. While I love to work with patients and do research, I knew I needed to prioritize my own health. As I did this, I realized it was the first time in my life I had ever made a commitment like this to myself and had communicated it to those around me. This was not easy for me, but it was incredibly important.

Of course, we can't control or change every source of stress in our lives. This is where the practice of mindfulness and meditation can help. Mindfulness simply means bringing our attention to what is occurring in the present moment, both externally and internally, and developing a willingness within ourselves to accept what we find. This helps to guide us away from getting bogged down in regrets of the past or fears and worries of the future, both of which can be a major source of stress. One of the things I like most about mindfulness is that it can be practiced at any time and in any place, and you can often feel the benefits of doing so immediately.

Meditating is like a formal practice of mindfulness, and setting aside time specifically for this purpose can be a very effective tool to manage stress in our lives. What I have found is that it's not always the challenge of a situation that creates the stress we experience, but rather our thoughts and perceptions about the situation. Meditation can help us notice our thoughts, and that allows us to redefine our responses to the challenges that arise. The bottom line here is that while we don't always have control over the events that arise in our lives, through mindfulness, meditation, and other stress management techniques that we'll discuss in chapter 5, we do have a choice in how we'll respond to stressors.

Sleep Hygiene

The phrase *sleep hygiene* refers to the quantity and quality of sleep you get each night and how this relates to your overall health. Believe it or not, one-third of adults report having difficulty sleeping, including trouble falling asleep, staying asleep, or waking far too early. Study after study has shown the correlation between inferior sleep and poor health outcomes.[3] What's more, as the population ages, the public health risks go up.[4] The upside is that the scientific community has the knowledge and understanding today to guide and support patients in achieving optimal sleep.

If poor sleep is an ongoing issue for you, know that you are not alone. I used to dread bedtime. It meant hours of tossing, turning, and worrying. Then came the MS diagnosis, and I found myself eagerly accepting prescriptions for sleep agents. The meds served two purposes: finally I was sleeping, and it also afforded a respite from the anxiety of my MS-controlled life, which felt like a bag of rocks. I found over time, however, that although I was sleeping eight to nine hours with these sleep aids, the character of sleep was poor, a kind of pseudo sleep that was robbing me of the health benefits of normal sleep and leaving me groggy and in a fog all day. Worse, when I woke up, I still had all the unresolved problems I had gone to bed with.

The other issue that quickly arose was my increasing tolerance to many of these drugs, which meant I needed larger doses or to switch to different classes of sleeping pills. Although the pharmaceutical industry denies these hypnotic agents are addictive, I disagree. Even if there is not a "physical" dependence, sleep is a psychosocial and emotional process, and one can grow dependent in those arenas, making it a burdensome task to try tapering off these medications.

Today I consider myself an advanced sleeper, but it took some hard lessons to get to where I am today. I am eager to share all of those with you so that you too can reap the remarkable benefits of a healthy sleep practice. The payoff is invaluable, particularly for someone who has suffered compromised quality of life with a sleep disorder over an extended period of time. Night after night of restful, recuperative sleep is indeed top-notch medicine, equated with fewer sick days, maintaining a healthy weight, reduced risk of diabetes and heart disease, less stress, better mood, and clear thinking, to name just a few.[5] Good sleep is something we can all achieve with a little planning and commitment, and we'll dive into how to do it in chapter 6.

Pulling back to look at the whole lifestyle medicine wheel for a moment, we can see how each spoke influences the others. When it comes to sleep, for example, nutrition, physical movement, and stress management create an environment that makes good sleep hygiene easier to achieve. With each positive change in lifestyle behavior, you can expect to feel the ripple effect through the entire wheel.

Substance Intake

There are a range of substances aside from food and medicine that we ingest, of course, and studies over the last few decades have shown that many of them are highly detrimental to our overall health and well-being. Naturally, then, it would follow that I advocate taking a good look at what kinds of substances you ingest and determining if they are consistent with your goal of achieving optimal health. What may surprise you is that in addition to familiar detrimental substances such as tobacco and alcohol, I also include the vast array of vitamins and supplements that are widely marketed as "healthy" in my list of substances we need to reevaluate.

Smoking

Most people know that there's no lifestyle behavior more harmful than smoking. Even with decreases over the past couple of decades, smoking is still a leading cause of preventable deaths in the United States.[6] Beyond the obvious lung cancer and heart disease connection, smoking contributes to other poor outcomes like stroke, diabetes, emphysema, chronic bronchitis, increased risk of tuberculosis, and autoimmune diseases. Indeed, it can affect nearly every part of your body.

In 1964, surgeon general Dr. Luther Terry presented the case that clearly spelled out tobacco's detrimental health effects supported by more than 7,000 studies.[7] Despite this condemning evidence, it took until 1993 for smoking to be banned from all hospitals in the United States.[8] This decision to universally remove tobacco use from health-care settings was a critically important change that correlated with a much wider shift in societal norms. Anti-smoking policy began to be implemented by state and local governments, businesses, schools, churches, and ultimately restaurants and bars. Undoubtedly, these restrictions coupled with higher taxes on tobacco products served to dramatically reduce smoking in the United States. Today the CDC reports nearly 14 percent of the population are active smokers—this is a far cry from a peak of 42 percent in 1964.[9] Despite this significant decline in tobacco use, however, cigarette smoking still accounts for a half million deaths in the United States per year. Smokers can expect to die ten years earlier than nonsmokers.[10] If you still smoke, I will offer some tips for quitting later in the book.

Drinking

Unlike smoking, alcohol still enjoys a largely positive public image, and is a much more acceptable and often celebrated practice. Raising a glass for a toast or drinking at a football game, a wedding, or a night out with the girls feels normal—alcohol consumption is expected, and abstaining can be isolating, even humiliating. In reality, excessive alcohol consumption contributes to heart disease, stroke, liver disease, cancer, dementia, and mental health issues like depression and anxiety.[11]

Just like the messaging we get around diet and food, there can be some confusion about whether consuming alcohol is beneficial. For instance, there has been some highly publicized research suggesting that red wine may afford some cardiovascular benefit, but you can actually get those same benefits from simply eating red grapes. While some research suggests that drinking wine might increase your HDL (the good cholesterol), there is no doubt that exercise can also do this. The

American Heart Association, contrary to what many people think, does *not* recommend drinking wine for improved heart health. The danger to your health that alcohol presents, along with the potential to destroy relationships, families, and lives, far outweighs the positives of supposed "health benefits" or social norms.

Vitamins and Supplements

Lastly, in many lifestyle medicine practices, discussions about substances are confined to smoking and drinking. I know that most of you reading this do not smoke, and some do not drink alcohol, so you may be tempted to skip this section. However, I would urge you to read it, because in my practice I also discuss with patients their use of vitamins and supplements, and how they, too, can be detrimental to your health if not used properly. This is a contentious topic, but I'll share why I feel this way in chapter 7.

Social Connection

You may be surprised to learn that spending time with friends and loved ones can be powerful medicine, but the facts are that those among us who remain isolated and lonely are at greater risk of chronic diseases like heart disease, obesity, stroke, pulmonary disease, and diabetes.[12]

One of my favorite anecdotes that is evidential of this comes from journalist Dan Buettner, who coined the term "blue zones" to refer to communities around the world where folks live longer, including Sardinia, Italy; Okinawa, Japan; and Loma Linda, California. Buettner has spent a lot of time learning about the daily habits of these people and noted a common thread of deep human bonds in each of these communities. He describes a custom in Okinawa called a *moai* (pronounced mo-eye), in which at a very young age, a small group of children are brought together in a ceremonial fashion and told they will always be there for one another, forever connected. The idea behind this practice is to have a built-in, lifelong support system through life's inevitable challenges as well as a group to share in the periods of joy. Many moai members reach old age together as a group, with astounding levels of health and well-being.[13]

Social connection can also affect the other spokes on the wheel. For instance, I often teach my patients the importance of fostering relationships with people who will support healthy choices in their lives. In other words, don't go on that lunch date with the friend who pressures you to order that big piece of chocolate cake for dessert. That friend may be a great choice for another type of social outing, but learning to surround yourself with the right people at the right time can help you achieve your overall goals.

I see this in my own practice when I hold a group support meeting. I may have eight patients who attend a group, all with a common set of goals. They may all be diabetics seeking to improve their outcomes. They often talk about how family and friends are not supportive, which makes it that much harder. These groups serve as our local moai, and I witness how these relationships foster positive outcomes. I see these patients begin to meet up for walks, share recipes, talk to one another about what's going on in their personal lives, and ultimately become lifelong friends. We'll discuss all the ways we can engage with community to not only boost our own well-being but also the health of those around us in chapter 8.

A Future You

As we come to the end of this lifestyle medicine overview, I want you to do a little mental exercise with me. I want you to imagine a set of identical twins. While these twins have the same genes, their daily habits and routines are totally different.

The first twin makes choices that he knows will benefit his health: he enjoys hiking and does so regularly with friends; he has made agreements at work that limit his stress; he doesn't smoke and rarely drinks; and he fills up his plate at mealtimes with whole plant-based foods.

The second twin didn't intend to make unhealthy choices, but over time he slipped into very different habits than his sibling—a diet with sugary drinks, processed foods, high-fat animal products, and a job that keeps him stressed and sitting in front of a computer until late in the evening. For this twin, exercise feels like a chore, and it's easier to veg at home in front of the TV than organize an outing with friends and family. His recent diagnosis of prediabetes carries a hefty load of guilt and is further eroding his self-confidence.

From a genetic standpoint, these twins are the same—and yet their health, happiness, and longevity have completely diverged.

Now imagine a "future you," a version of yourself that is identical but has made different choices and is enjoying different outcomes. Let go of any shame and guilt you might have about the past, and be completely OK with wherever you are right now in terms of your own health and well-being. Now is the time you can start making changes for that future you—for your health, longevity, and happiness—and the rest of this book will show you exactly how to do it.

Step by Step

In the next few chapters, we'll dive into each spoke on the lifestyle medicine wheel. At the end of each chapter is a brief recap of key ideas plus step-by-step actions you can take to help you put the changes I will recommend into practice and undergo your own personal transformation in the process. To that aim, we will start here with a self-assessment. I believe that it's important to take some time to check in honestly with yourself and then physically write out a current assessment of where you are today. This will give you a baseline to measure your progress toward your goals, and consequently make them more obtainable. Remember, the ultimate goal here is to transform your life, and that will require looking at several different areas. I recommend picking up a notebook or journal especially for the purpose of writing about your own journey of transformation. Doing so can strengthen your resolve to make changes, and provide a way to look back and see how far you've already come on those days when it feels tough to stick with the changes.

Keep It Simple Review

The six spokes of the lifestyle medicine wheel that promote prevention and healing are:

1. Food—eat more plants

2. Exercise—play more

3. Stress—stay present

4. Sleep—rest well

5. Substances—thrive without

6. Connection—grow love

Self-Assessment

The best place to start this journey is with a written assessment of where you are today. This is very similar to what I would be asking you if you were a patient sitting in my office. Before you begin, please remember two things: First, it's important to be as honest as possible here; no one needs to see your answers but you, and the more honest you can be about the way things are, the better you can tailor your plan going forward. Second, do not use this tool as an opportunity for judgment or comparison. Wherever you are today is OK. The more you can look at your current state objectively, the more clarity and strength you can draw on to make lasting changes in your life. With those things in mind, let's get started.

1. Briefly summarize why you are seeking to transform your life.

2. Please list and describe what goals or ideal health outcomes you would like to achieve in the next year, five years, lifetime?

3. **Diet:** Record a food diary over at least a 48-hour period that is representative of what you typically eat, include at least one weekday and one weekend day. Once you record exactly what you are eating, review this objective information and ponder these questions:

> a. Do you feel satisfied after meals? Are you hungry between meals?
>
> b. Do you tend to overeat?
>
> c. How often do you consume animal products like meat, dairy, and eggs?
>
> d. Do you tend to skip meals? If so, why?
>
> e. What do you eat for snacks? What triggers snacking?
>
> f. How many times a week to do you eat out?
>
> g. Are most of the meals eaten at home consumed at the dinner table with family members?
>
> h. Do you experience cravings? If so, can you describe when they are heightened?

(For a simple chart to help you track this, see the food diary template in appendix A.)

4. **Exercise.** Do you exercise? If so, describe the physical activity. How many times per week do you exercise and for how long? How hard are you working when you exercise? Do you feel winded? What other movement are you doing right now? Are you engaged in weekly strength training exercises? What motivates you to exercise right now, if anything? Describe any limitations you feel.

5. **Stress**. How frequently do you feel overwhelmed or anxious? On a scale of 1 to 10, what is your current stress level? Can you identify the main source of your stress? Do you have any experience meditating? Do you practice daily prayer? If so, do you meditate or pray currently?

6. **Sleep.** How many hours of sleep do you get per night? Do you have trouble falling asleep? Are you able to stay asleep? How many times do you get up in the night? Do you watch screens before bed? Would you describe your sleep as deep and restful? What is your sleep environment like now? What are your presleep rituals? (See appendix B for a basic chart you can use to help you organize this information.)

7. **Substances.** List daily or weekly intake of any alcohol, smoking, recreational drugs, or supplements.

8. **Relationships**. Think of your circle of family, friends, colleagues, and acquaintances. In whom can you confide? How often do you feel lonely? Who is the biggest supporter of your health and well-being?

9. **Current Conditions**. List each chronic illness or condition for which you have been diagnosed and are being treated by your doctor along with all the medications and treatments you are taking for its management.

Diagnosis_____

Treatment_____

(Include any medicines, procedures, or supplements you are taking for this condition. Do this for each diagnosis if more than one.

When you've finished with your assessment, take a moment to congratulate yourself. You have just documented a comprehensive overview of where you stand today. You've taken an important step toward personal self-awareness and have begun your journey toward a healthier you.

The great value of this assessment is to bring awareness to each aspect of lifestyle so that as you read this book, you can note what changes you need to employ to improve from your baseline. Over time, you will have journaled your personal transformation: looking back in a year you will be surprised to see how much needed change you have welcomed into your life! Now that you have a basic picture of each of the spokes and how they come together as a whole practice, it's time to set this wheel in motion and begin your journey of personal transformation.

The Plant-Centered Plate

Let food be thy medicine and medicine be thy food.
—Hippocrates

Eight years into living with MS, I made the decision to switch to a set of healthy principles that I didn't even know were called lifestyle medicine at the time. The first of these was diet, and before I changed it, I thought it through very carefully. I had to; I was encountering a lot of opposition. This was back in the days before films like *Forks Over Knives* and other resources were widely available, so I was largely on my own.

My physicians warned me that it was irresponsible to wean myself off of the ten to twelve medications I was taking daily (and that were making my life unbearable) and solely manage my MS with an "unproven lifestyle change." Even my husband, also a physician, was concerned (remember, at the time I was flying in the face of the conventional wisdom about MS). But I am first and foremost a scientist, and the research was clear. I adopted a whole foods, plant-based diet because the overwhelming body of scientific literature pointed to those foods as the best diet for optimal health for all people. At that point, I knew I could not face a lifetime living as I was—with a huge pillbox, cane, diapers, and the other physical and psychological burdens of MS. I decided that I would do whatever I could to get a few years of quality life, even if it shortened my overall life span, by opting out of the conventional treatment that was meant to slow the progression of my disease. Of course,

I didn't know then what is crystal clear now—that the changes I was considering would improve my overall health and well-being, increase my longevity, *and* slow my MS in remarkable ways.

Looking back, I know now that this was the best decision I ever made, but I can also see that it was harder than it needed to be. That's because I made these significant changes to my diet without guidance from a health-care professional. That's a big part of the reason I spend so much time and energy getting this message out into the world. I want it to be easier for my patients—and for you. I sometimes feel like I've been given a secret key to demystify healthy eating and unlock how truly simple it can be—and I can't help but want to share it with everyone.

In my first consultations with patients, we spend a lot of time on the nutrition spoke of the lifestyle medicine wheel. There are a few reasons for this. First of all, *eating well feels good*, and it can quickly offset some of the pain and suffering I see in my patients when they first come in— sometimes in unexpected ways. For instance, you might be surprised at how much more energy you have as a result of giving up junk food. Because of this, looking at food first is a good way to kick-start a total lifestyle overhaul.

Second, since the medical establishment downplays the role of food in healing, most of my patients get some version of an aha moment with even just a little education on the subject. For example, when I share the overwhelming evidence of the benefits associated with consuming a primarily plant-based diet, patients are typically very eager to get started right away.

Lastly, another good reason to start with food is that there's no downside to the kind of simple advice I give my patients—no side effects, no complicated regimen to learn—and the upside is that eating in the way I'll describe actually benefits the whole body. For example, if you are eager to improve your diet because you have been recently diagnosed with rheumatoid arthritis (RA), eating in this way will help your RA, but it will also have the bonus effect of reducing your risk of heart disease, diabetes, and cancer.

Food for Life

The ideas introduced in this book are meant to be food for life. That is, we are not eating this way for a few months or a year; this is a lifelong venture. Because you are embarking on meaningful and lasting change, as you introduce small changes it's important to reinforce them daily, and soon they will become habits. I have no doubt you can do this, and I encourage you to enjoy the process and be kind to yourself when things don't go perfectly. Use any momentary lapses or setbacks as lessons to strengthen and grow. I'll offer more tips about how to do this as we move along. I would like to begin with a quote from Michael Pollan:

Eat food. Not too much. Mostly plants.[1]

When I read that and compared it to my extensive review of the medical research on nutrition, I thought, *Yep. That pretty much sums it up.* The only thing I'd quibble with is actually an added bonus for those of us choosing a plant-based diet . . . we really can't eat "too much." Most Americans do eat too much when it comes to the processed foods, meat, and dairy that we routinely pile on our plates. We certainly don't want to eat too much of those, so if you are opting to keep some animal protein in your diet, it's important to listen to Pollan's "not too much" advice. Plant-based foods are so rich in fiber that they simply take up too much real estate in your stomach to go overboard. These foods have tons of nutrients and few calories. It's the difference between eating 100 calories of broccoli (a whole plate or more) and 100 calories of steak, which translates to a few bites.

When I am asked the question, "Dr. Stancic, what should I eat to maintain maximum health?" The answer is simple: *Eat mostly plants.* How does this translate into building our plates? It means consuming a whole foods, plant-based diet. Every day, eat fruits, vegetables, whole grains, legumes, nuts, and seeds; eat few or no animal foods (including dairy and eggs); and avoid processed foods altogether, which I refer to as "foodstuffs." Foodstuffs are highly processed prepackaged items you can find in any grocery store: sugary cereals, chips, pastries, cookies, and the like. Many of these products have literally been made in a lab to be what food scientists call hyperpalatable. They are layered with sugar, salt, and fat in ways that trigger gut and brain biochemical signals that build irresistible cravings and even addiction.[2] With "eat mostly plants" as a rallying cry and overall directive, let's look at a simple plan for making this work for you.

Step 1: Eat More Plants

You may be lukewarm on the idea of a drastic change to your diet. Maybe the word *vegan* evokes radical, negative imagery for you—you certainly wouldn't be the only one. You might feel like you "should" change, but you're afraid you'll lose the joy of eating the things you love. You've probably seen friends or family members struggle with highly restrictive diets, often giving up because they are unsustainable—and you may have a history of doing this yourself. As you can imagine, adding a bunch of rules, restrictions, and protocols to your everyday life can start to feel as daunting as the chronic disease treatment regimen you might be trying to escape. So let me say this: It's no use running yourself ragged trying to keep up a "perfect" health plan; there's no point in transforming your life into one of misery and limitation. We're after well-being and joy here—that's what will truly sustain you through inevitable challenges and setbacks.

To that end, allow me to offer a gentle shift in mindset. Typically, when you ask someone what they ate for dinner, they respond with something like, "I had chicken/fish/steak." No one says, "I had broccoli/asparagus/sweet potato," because we don't think like that. In our society, animal protein is the main event, and the veggies are the afterthought or "sides." This can mean that a heaping plate of veggies and fruits can still feel like a partial meal at the beginning. It's no fun to feel like something is missing, so one of the first and easiest ways to change your diet is to keep it all on the plate but switch up the proportions. I once had a patient throw up his hands in my office and say, "I can't do this. I love steak, and there's no way I can give up my special steak dinner once a week." And I get it.

While I would love for you to go to a 100 percent plant-based diet, I realize that the thought of this is scary for some people. If that describes you, let's start instead by reorganizing your plate.

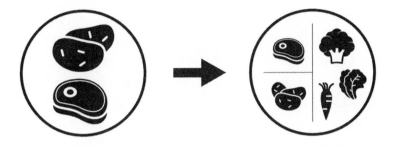

In this way, we go from a plate full of meat and dairy with one potato, to a plate where three-quarters of the foods are plant-based. A smaller portion of steak, a potato with a dash of salt/pepper and maybe some herbs like chives or parsley, and a half plate of *colorful* vegetables like carrots, broccoli, asparagus, zucchini, and mushrooms. (Side note: While mushrooms are regularly included as vegetables in culinary circles, scientifically speaking, they are a fungus. Regardless of where they are classified, they are an excellent food source, packed with antioxidants, vitamins, and minerals.)

Eat the Rainbow

When we "eat the rainbow," we enjoy plants of all colors. The vibrant hues indicate what's inside: each one has a different combination of powerful antioxidants and phytonutrients, which are key players in maintaining an anti-inflammatory environment in our cells and in turn serve to preserve our overall well-being and reduce our risk of chronic disease.

For example, lycopene is responsible for the tomato's vibrant red color. The blueberry gets its purple pigment from a formidable phytonutrient called anthocyanin. It really doesn't matter what the antioxidant is called—the valuable lesson here is that by filling your plate with plants of differing colors, you get a variety of health-promoting nutrients as a result. With so many options, it's easy to keep your plate interesting by changing it up with the seasons and ensuring that you are getting a variety of phytonutrients every time you sit down to enjoy a meal.

With this step, you're not only eating fewer calories on a more generous plate of food, you are also eating smarter. Smart foods grow from the earth and are rich in phytonutrients and fiber. The healthiest foods we can eat all have fiber. And fiber is found only in plants; there is no fiber in animals or their by-products. Fiber reduces cholesterol, normalizes blood sugar, keeps the bowels regular, offers satiety, reduces our risk of heart disease, diabetes, and cancer, and on and on. But the most important reason fiber-rich diets are essential to our overall well-being may lie in our gut. I am referring to one of the hottest research areas in clinical medicine today, the gut microbiome.

Protect Your Gut

The gut microbiome (gut flora) is an ecosystem of microorganisms that live in our lower gastrointestinal tract. This vast population of microbes surpasses several trillion cells, and it serves many important functions in our overall health and well-being. Researchers are working to better understand and characterize the gut flora and its implications in health.[3]

Working away unseen, gut bacteria can help strengthen your immune system, maintain a healthy weight, and reduce the risk of diabetes, cancer, and heart disease.[4] There is even evidence suggesting that having a healthy microbiome can reduce the risk of dementia.[5] Conversely, an imbalance in gut flora can lead to health problems in every part of the body, including heart disease, cancer, autoimmune disease, and even psychiatric disorders. Healthy gut flora is diverse gut flora, and one in which the "good bugs" outnumber the "bad bugs." The best way to get this essential diversity and enrichment of favorable bugs?[6] Fiber.

A recent Italian study compared the gut flora of MS patients with and without a plant-enriched diet and found a difference in the quality and diversity of the gut microbiome, as well as a corresponding decrease in relapse rates and disability in patients who ate more plants.[7] This study may help vindicate Dr. Roy Swank, who for decades was criticized for suggesting a low-fat plant-based diet could serve to better manage MS.

In the end, what you put on your plate affects the bugs in your gut, and the bugs in your gut in turn produce chemical signals that in the case of MS may either stimulate the immune response to attack the brain and spinal cord or signal the immune system to stop the onslaught.[8] This process may apply to the genesis of all chronic diseases. Consume fiber in the form of whole plant-based foods, and good things happen.

Step 2: Eat Enough to Feel Satisfied

Did you know that the average human needs to consume about four pounds of food every day to feel full and satisfied? Of course, four pounds of apples, blueberries, sweet potatoes, arugula, barley, tomatoes, quinoa, and black beans looks and feels very different than four pounds of steak, bacon, cake, and cheese. Many of my patients get excited when I show them how much food they can eat when they're eating mostly plants. We're so often told that "healthy eating" means eating less, but in this case four pounds really looks and feels like a lot. I want to make sure they're eating enough to feel full and happy, and very often eating more plants means losing weight. Why? Because there are fewer calories per pound of food, plus lots of fiber, and tons of phytonutrients.

Does this mean I want you to weigh your food, count calories, or set up a point system to monitor intake? No. Your food diary can be helpful, especially at the beginning of making dietary changes, and I'm including a way to do that in the appendix at the end of this book. For myself and my patients, I have found that the kind of restrictive weighing and measuring (which is often associated with dieting and diet culture) robs us of the joy of food as a sustaining, healing, health-giving force. Keep it simple, keep it enjoyable.

Remember, *eat mostly plants*. That's it.

Step 3: Try a Variety of Foods

You might have heard that potatoes aren't healthy, or that fruit has too much sugar so you should limit your intake. When my patients ask, "What plants should I eat?" My response couldn't be simpler: "All of them." Potatoes and fruit in their whole form have tons of fiber and nutrients (not french fries and fruit roll-ups, of course). The key, again, is variety—bringing as many different whole fruits and veggies to your plate as possible over time.

I don't know very many doctors who go grocery shopping with their patients, but I do. It helps me to get a firsthand look at a patient's beliefs and habits around food, and it can be an eye-opening experience for both of us. In terms of expanding variety, we break it down into a few steps. First, start with plants you know you already love. Potatoes, corn, apples, spinach, and green beans? Great, let's increase the amount and frequency of those. Put double in the cart. One patient realized that even though she really liked apples, she only ate an apple once a week. On a shopping trip, we picked up seven apples, and she planned to put them on her counter and eat one every day.

Once you master eating more of what you love, try adding things you haven't had in some time. Before her next shopping trip, I asked my patient to come up with something she hadn't tried in a while—cauliflower, asparagus, or artichokes maybe. This is a way to rediscover things that have dropped off your list of preferred foods. Typically, a patient will get excited about at least one of these, adding it to their regular rotation.

Third, you want to tackle foods that are on your "hate" list. For this patient, it was lima beans. We found a recipe that included other ingredients and spices she knew she liked, and the lima beans became tolerable.

Finally, trying foods you've never had before may be the hardest part to building your plant repertoire, but expanding your options keeps things interesting and provides you with an even greater range of nutrients. Many of my patients suffer from food neophobia, meaning they are afraid to try new or unfamiliar foods. Evolutionarily speaking, this makes sense, as it protected us from possibly consuming a toxic food in times past—but because the twenty-first-century global economy gives us access to foods from all corners of the earth, we have a unique opportunity to sample different cultures' ingredients and dishes that previous generations didn't have. This allows our options to become markedly enriched and varied. As you can see, I love diversity!

To recap, here's how to build your plant-based repertoire:

1. Increase the amount and frequency of plants you already enjoy: "I love apples, so I will eat an apple a day."

2. Revisit plants you haven't tried in some time: "I had cauliflower at a wedding in 2010, and it wasn't terrible."

3. Give plants you hate a second chance: "I hated lima beans when I was a kid, but I'm willing to try them again."

4. Try something new: "I've never tried mango before, but I'm willing to try it in a cabbage mango coleslaw recipe for my tacos."

Taking a more adventurous and inquisitive approach to food can expand the variety on our plates very quickly. Whenever you find yourself getting bored or feeling limited or deprived, check out a new cookbook, cooking blog, or chef's account on social media. Try to incorporate different types of cuisines and ingredients. Eating a wide variety of foods is also a great example for any children in your household. Research tells us that children may need to be exposed to a food at least eight times in order to change their preference.[9] Keep offering a variety of foods, without comment and without shaming, and show your kids how much you enjoy eating the rainbow, and you'll expand their palate as well.

Choose Real Food

As you make these changes, I want you to be sure to choose real food. What do I mean by real food? Well, one of my favorite litmus tests for "real food" is to imagine my own great-grandmother and what she would do if someone handed her a plastic-wrapped, neon-colored fruit roll-up. She wouldn't even recognize it as food, let alone fruit, and she wouldn't know how to eat it.

Real food does not come from a factory or a lab; it comes from nature. We want to shop for, prepare, and eat food that is in its natural, whole state or as close to it as possible. For some people, this poses an immediate challenge. *What if I'm not a good cook? How do I know what's ripe or will taste good in the produce section?* Furthermore, some Americans live in what are known as food deserts with limited access to fresh foods (but meanwhile convenience stores with chips and candy bars lurk at every gas station). The good news is, with a little planning and a few basic guidelines, you can expand your ability to shop for and prepare whole foods. If you already love to cook, all the better—many of my patients discover great joy by finding new and innovative ways to bulk up the plants in their favorite recipes.

The Whole Foods, Plant-Based Pyramid

Here's another simple way to think about the essential elements of a whole foods, plant-based diet: my version of the plant-powered pyramid can be seen on the next page.

Fruits and Vegetables

The lifestyle medicine prescription encourages consumption of *all* fruits and vegetables, without restriction. I'm often asked, "Can diabetics eat fruit?" Absolutely. A massive study which included half a million participants followed over several years found that among those who were diabetes-free at the start, eating fruit every day *reduced* the risk of diabetes by 12 percent. In those who already had diabetes, consuming fruit regularly resulted in a 17 percent reduced risk of dying of any cause and

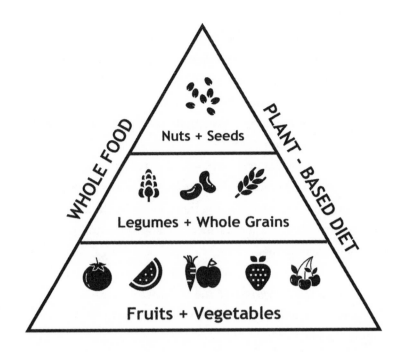

as much as a 28 percent lower risk of developing a diabetes-related complication.[10] This study puts that question to rest once and for all. Fruit consumption should be encouraged in all people, including diabetics. Bear in mind, however, that I mean whole fruit, not fruit juice. Without the fiber that would be in a piece of whole fruit, fruit juice packs too much of a sugar punch. Whole fruit is always a better choice. An apple a day does keep the doctor away!

Legumes and Whole Grains

Legumes include beans, lentils, and peas. They are a great source of fiber and protein, and they are far less expensive than animal protein per ounce. Interestingly, a cross-cultural, worldwide study conducted by the World Health Organization showed that eating more legumes meant longer lives for the elderly, regardless of their ethnicity.[11] Remember the blue zones discussed earlier with extraordinary rates of longevity? We can all emulate the Okinawans, who feast on generous amounts of miso and tofu (traditional foods based on soybeans), and the Sardinians, whose plates are enriched with chickpeas, cannellini beans, and lentils.

Whole grains include oats, brown rice, barley, quinoa, buckwheat, wild rice, and millet. It's best to eat these as close to their natural form as possible. When choosing whole grains that are packaged, read the labels. It's not uncommon to find a box of cereal that is labeled "whole grain," but when you read the label, you find that it is much more like a foodstuff than real food.[12] When purchasing whole grains that have some element of processing, choose those that have the shortest list of ingredients (whole grain should be first), and shoot for at least four grams of fiber per serving.

Unprocessed or unrefined whole grains are composed of three parts or layers: the bran, the germ, and the endosperm. The bran is the fiber and nutrient-rich outer layer, while the germ, also rich in nutrients, including protein, is the inner seedling. Refining a grain removes both of these precious layers, leaving behind the endosperm alone, which is primarily starch or carbohydrate. The refining process strips this otherwise food treasure of all of its valuable gems, including fiber, protein, vitamins, phytonutrients, and elements like magnesium and zinc. The bran plays a key role in slowing the absorption of glucose and averting sharp blood sugar spikes. Without question, whole grains improve our blood sugar.

Eating real whole grains can have a positive effect on inflammation, too. One study followed 40,000 postmenopausal women over a period of seventeen years, assessing the role whole grain intake would play in inflammatory disease. They were looking at autoimmune diseases like rheumatoid arthritis, ulcerative colitis, Crohn's disease, type 1 diabetes mellitus, and inflammatory diseases like chronic obstructive pulmonary disease, and asthma. They found a 35 percent reduction in risk of death secondary to inflammatory disease in those who consumed the highest intake of whole grains.[13]

Of course, it's difficult to talk about whole grains in today's food climate without addressing two big contemporary issues—gluten and carbs—but I'll address these later in the chapter (my answers may surprise you!).

Nuts and Seeds

At the top of the pyramid sit nuts and seeds, which are great sources of good fat, fiber, protein, vitamins, minerals, and other important things like antioxidants and phytosterols. They're at the top of the pyramid, though, because they should make up a smaller portion of our overall diet (we don't want to sit mindlessly in front of the television with a bowl full of cashews, because they are rich in fat and can pack on a lot of calories). Eat nuts and seeds sparingly and as an add-on, like a garnish. I'll throw a handful of walnuts onto my oatmeal, add some cashews to a veggie stir-fry, or spoon some pine nuts or pumpkin seeds onto a salad to add texture and crunch.

Restock Your Pantry with Fresh, Wholesome Foods

A good place to begin is in your pantry. Noted chef and government nutrition policy advisor Sam Kass recommends a three-step process: first, purge your pantry (while still keeping a few treats on hand, if desired); second, reorganize to make fresh food more visible and available; and third, prep foods ahead of time so they'll be easier to cook with later.[14] We'll cover meal planning and grocery shopping a little later on.

Some people enjoy the challenge of going through their entire pantry and gleefully tossing whatever isn't working for them anymore, and if that's the way you want to go, make a holiday out of it and have a good time! But bear in mind that you definitely don't need to tackle everything in there at once. A major pantry purge isn't always the most practical approach, especially when you're sticking to a budget. For those who want to ease in, find one food or category to review and take a hard look at it. For example, breakfast: if you often eat cold cereal in the morning, take out all the cereals you have in your pantry. Read the labels and see how many ingredients you recognize versus how many you don't. If you're surprised by how many grams of sugar are listed on the label or how many chemicals and preservatives you see, toss it, and replace it with whole fruit and a bowl of oatmeal. Then, as time allows, check out other items in your pantry. Maybe you'll find many of the foods you have, like canned beans, dried lentils, and whole grains such as quinoa and farro, are good to keep. But if there's a lot of processed food in there, do what you can to weed those items out.

Once you've taken stock of all the food that's available to you at home, put it away where you can see it and grab it easily. This simple step can be life-changing. If we're talking about fresh foods, so often we don't eat fruits and veggies because we don't see them first. The drawers at the bottom of the fridge stay closed, and the fresh food spoils before we remember to eat it. In my own kitchen, I have switched up the storage in my fridge, so that I keep all the condiments in the bottom drawers. I fill up the visible shelves with vegetables, fruit, and nondairy beverages. The same goes for my pantry. I keep plant staples like beans and whole grains front and center and put any treats as well as nuts and seeds in opaque containers out of the way. Also, I suggest keeping a big bowl of fruit on your countertop for easy access, and finding one or two simple vegetable soups that you love that are easily adaptable. That way, any leftover veggies can go in the pot before they go bad.

Finally, prep foods so they're ready to go later, and if you need to go shopping, bring a list and stick to it. When I shop with my patients, they are often surprised by a few habits I live by. Grocery stores are set up to prey on our worst instincts when it comes to food. Ever notice that the produce section is almost always on the right? That's because most people are right-handed and tend to turn that way first. That may seem like a good thing, but store layout designers know that once we've visited the produce section, with its vibrant colors and healthy fruits and vegetables, we'll feel upbeat, hungry, and righteous about our healthy choices, so we'll be primed to stay in the store longer and say yes to a cart full of meat, dairy, and foodstuffs (which have the highest profit margins in the food industry).[15] These impulse buys are bad for our health and our wallet. So when I go into the store, the first thing I do is turn to the left and pick up offerings such as whole grain bread, peanut butter, almond milk, nuts, a bounty of grains; oats, brown rice and barley, and spices like turmeric, cinnamon, and cumin from the middle aisles (avoiding the cereal, chips, cookies, and soda). I will also swing through and grab some dried or canned beans or frozen vegetables and fruit, but my real destination is the produce section, where I fill up my cart with a variety of delicious plants last. This seems like a simple thing, but it can have a huge impact on the way you shop.

I know that the grocery budget is a concern for many, and I know there are certainly cases where processed foods are less expensive than whole and healthy ones, but there are resources available that can help. For example, there are several chefs and authors who have addressed this very issue like Darshana Thacker, chef and culinary program manager at Forks Over Knives, who describes a $1.50 a day and $5 a day healthy whole foods, plant-based meal plan.[16]

Here are a few more suggestions:

- Try bulk bin shopping; a wide variety of beans and grains are generally available and at reasonably low prices.

- Check out the frozen section. Often high-quality produce is available at good prices.

- Look for services that offer blemished produce. Often shoppers are looking for "picture-perfect" food, but there are companies that sell foods that have spots or minor damage for bargain prices.

- Consider joining a CSA or Community Supported Agriculture; in this way, you are actually buying a local farm share. Members receive a box of produce on average once a week during the growing season. This approach is much cheaper when you are buying directly from the farmer, and your produce is also much fresher as it is local.

• Join or form a buying club. Food distributors often offer wholesale prices not just to stores but to groups that buy in sufficient quantities.

Meal Planning

Many people find it helpful when undertaking a dietary change to plan their meals out in advance. Several patients have told me that when they stumbled, it was often because they didn't have a plan for what they were going to eat on a particular day, and then something came up and threw them offtrack. We all know how quick and accessible processed foods are, and this can be an easy trap to fall into if you run late at work and get home and realize you didn't plan a healthy meal. Having a plan, and even preparing meals in advance as much as possible, can help you avoid this pitfall. It can also help you bring variety to your plate as you can creatively brainstorm what you'd like to eat for the week.

Here's what a typical few days of planning might look like for me:

Day 1

Note: Water is important! I make sure to drink water with all my meals and throughout the day.

6 a.m.: Breakfast: Bowl of oatmeal with 1 heaping tablespoon of ground flaxseed and cinnamon with a handful of walnuts, bowl of blueberries and raspberries, and cup of black coffee.

10 a.m.: Midmorning snack: An apple with a few almonds.

12:30 p.m.: Lunch: A bowl with four bean chili served over quinoa, roasted brussels sprouts, beets, and sliced avocado, with fresh cilantro and lime juice squeezed over top.

4 p.m.: Midafternoon snack: White bean hummus with slices of red pepper.

6:30 p.m.: Chickpeas with potatoes, peas in tomato sauce (fricassee) served over brown rice with a salad of romaine lettuce, avocados, cucumbers, radishes, and red onion.

Day 2

6 a.m.: Breakfast: Oats with chia seeds soaked overnight in almond milk with nutmeg and cinnamon, a sliced pear, cup of black coffee.

10 a.m.: Midmorning snack: Orange slices.

12:30 p.m.: Lunch: Sandwich of whole grain bread with hummus, sliced apple, sprouts, and pickles with a side kale salad with dry cranberries and pumpkin seeds dressed with balsamic vinaigrette.

4 p.m.: Midafternoon snack: Peach with pistachios.

6:30 p.m.: Grilled portobello mushrooms with sautéed onions, Cuban black beans served over brown rice, steamed yuca (cassava) dressed with mojo (lime juice, dash of olive oil, garlic, and shallots) with a spinach salad, cherry tomatoes and red onion.

Day 3

6 a.m.: Breakfast: Whole grain toast with almond butter and a sliced apple, cup of black coffee.

10 a.m.: Midmorning snack: Pineapple chunks with handful of almonds.

12:30 p.m.: Lunch: Pasta fagioli soup, slice of whole grain sourdough bread, arugula, and watermelon.

4 p.m.: Midafternoon snack: A couple of plums.

6:30 p.m.: Roasted cauliflower tacos served with guacamole and a red cabbage/mango slaw over a bed of watercress.

I hope this little example gets you thinking about how you can plan your own meals over the course of a few days or preferably an entire week.

A Note about "Success" and "Failure"

My own journey has been far from perfect. For the first several years of my lifestyle treatment plan, I continued to experience periods when my worst neurological MS symptoms returned. The first one came at around six months into my self-devised lifestyle treatment, and my doctor at the time was blunt, telling me "you brought this on yourself." It was terrible. I started to question what I was doing, but something pushed me to keep going. My amazing husband helped me see that what my doctor was calling failure might actually be part of a bigger success. He saw that there were small things marking my progress: I could stay up past the evening news, and I had a little bit more optimism even though I had come off of antidepressant medication. Things were going in the right direction. As far as the MS was concerned, I wasn't sure where my journey would take me or what exactly future success would entail, but I knew deep down that I needed to keep going.

Two years into my improved lifestyle management plan, I felt confident that things were really getting better. The MS exacerbations went from occurring every three to six months to maybe one a year; and when they happened, they were milder and I could recover more quickly. I never say that I've been cured of MS. Success for me is a journey, not a destination. If I decided tomorrow that I was going to sit on the couch and eat cheeseburgers, I know I would regress immediately. Even now, I can feel it when I don't get enough sleep, or carry extra stress. Rather than those things scaring me or feeling guilty about them, however, I thank them. Because my health is back on track, I can feel certain that any pain or fatigue is an effective warning for me, a reminder that I need an extra dose of self-care.

Be gentle with yourself. New students of meditation, for example, are often told that should they miss a meditation session, fall asleep during meditation, or even stop meditating altogether for a time, they should remember that they can always "begin again." Each "failure," therefore, is simply an invitation to begin again.

With each of these six lifestyle changes, and especially diet and nutrition, you're never going to get it "100 percent right." There will be days when you're superbusy and you feel like you don't have time to prepare a delicious salad, or days when you're tired, or sick, and don't feel motivated to cook for yourself. That's OK; just pick up where you left off, and try to be as consistent as you can overall. The goal is that you'll have a healthy relationship with food and you'll be excited to eat in a way that feels good for your body and your mind. Does this mean you'll never eat a piece of cake again? No. You'll find yourself at birthday parties, holiday parties, and weddings, and it's OK if you want to have a treat now and again. Communing over food is wonderful, and it doesn't happen for the majority of our meals. Allow yourself to enjoy food and the company of others, and I'll bet you'll look forward to returning to your routine of nutritious food that you've prepared for yourself once the event is over. It's not about "succeeding" or "failing"; it's about consistency, and routine, and returning to healthy habits when we deviate from them—without judgment or guilt.

Questions and Challenges

In addition to seeing patients at my lifestyle medicine practice, I regularly give lectures around the country about the benefits of lifestyle medicine. Because of the complicated history in our society between profit-driven diet fads, a wealth of misinformation, as well as a genuine desire from people to know the truth about what constitutes a healthy diet, I wanted to share answers to the most common questions and challenges I hear from my patients and in my travels. I know from experience that many of you reading this will have these same questions, too.

Question: Is it healthier to be gluten-free?

For the overwhelming majority of the population, no, it isn't healthier to be gluten-free. Gluten is a beneficial protein found in many grains.

Patients with celiac disease (1 percent of the population) should certainly cut out gluten, but unless you have been diagnosed with this disease, cutting gluten from your diet is likely unnecessary and often unhelpful, as doing so can restrict otherwise healthy options from finding their way onto your plate. In other words, I have had patients tell me how they chose less healthy options in order to avoid something that contained gluten, even though they don't have celiac disease. To me, this is an example of how marketing can falsely influence our understanding of foods and their effect on health. Many of these gluten-free foods are prepackaged, processed foodstuffs that are actually harmful to your health. There is a category of patients that fall under a designation called "gluten intolerant or sensitive," these patients report subjective improvement in symptoms when they exclude gluten from their diet. This is a minority.

Question: Aren't carbs bad for you?

Here, again, we find that advertising and diet fads have created confusion for many people when it comes to carbs, which are not inherently bad for you. In fact, carbohydrates should be bountiful in your diet, as long as they are from whole foods. What we want to avoid are processed foods like cookies, cakes, donuts, bagels, etc. I don't call these carbs—I call them foodstuffs. Grouping or labeling foods as macronutrients, like carbohydrate, fat, and protein, confuses dietary advice—one might equate a cookie with a sweet potato, when in fact the carbs in sweet potatoes are nothing like the carbs in cookies. Patients often tell me they avoid bread and pasta because they are carbs, while of course choosing a highly refined and processed bread would be categorized as a foodstuff and a whole grain bread or whole wheat pasta would be acceptable additions to your healthy plant-based table. I advocate discarding this type of thinking entirely and keeping it simple: choose real foods, mostly plants, and eat the rainbow.

Question: Does adopting this lifestyle mean the end to dining out?

When we eat out at restaurants, we lose control of the ingredient list. Keep in mind the chef is creating a dish that will appeal to the vast majority of people primed to enjoy foods that are rich in sugar, salt, and fat. With that said, this doesn't mean you can't choose primarily plants when you are eating at a restaurant. For example, begin with a colorful salad, then order main dishes such as whole wheat pasta primavera, vegetarian paella, avocado/cucumber sushi, or even cobble together two yummy veggie side dishes. You can even ask to alter an existing option on the menu by asking the waiter to exclude the cheese or meat from a main dish (e.g., spaghetti without the meatballs). A few years ago, I was invited to my sister in law's fiftieth birthday party at a steak house in New York City. When it came time to place my order, I very politely explained to the waitress that I ate a plant-based diet and asked if she would suggest a suitable order. She smiled and said, "Our chef also eats a plant-based diet and he will be happy to prepare something for you." I was presented with a trio of perfectly prepared vegetables. It was delicious! Everyone at the table complimented my choice and even asked to sample it. So yes, you can eat out but be mindful about how frequently you choose to do so. It is almost always best to prepare our own meals at home.

Challenge: Help! I'm addicted to foodstuffs!

The hyperpalatable foodstuffs we've discussed pack a double unhealthy punch: they lack phytonutrients, fiber, vitamins, minerals, etc., plus they have additives beyond sugar, salt, and fat that make them truly hazardous, such as preservatives, chemicals, and food colorings. Not only are these foodstuffs designed (visually and chemically) to be incredibly appealing, but we are often bombarded with advertisements selling them at every turn, making it even more of a challenge to keep them off our plates.

Swimming upstream against marketing and taste-enhanced food-stuffs can be difficult, but it can be done! Here are some suggestions: First, limit your exposure to food advertising. Avoid the center aisles of the grocery store. Do a pantry purge of these items already in your home, if you can. As Sam Kass suggests, discard "anything with sugar in any of its many forms—high-fructose corn syrup, fruit juice concentrate, cane sugar, and so on—as one of the first few ingredients," or anything that contains a bunch of stuff you can't pronounce.

Challenge: I don't have time to cook.

The prospect of adding a lot of cooking time can be overwhelming. Likewise, foodstuffs are often cheap, quick, and easy (even though they are horrible for your overall health). I've found the best way to eliminate them is to have healthy alternatives on hand that have the same qualities.

Set aside some time on a Saturday or Sunday afternoon to make big batches of grains and legumes that can go into fast meals throughout the week. Cut up vegetables and fruits you love so they are easy to grab and go. Find a few emergency meal starters in the frozen food section, carefully reading the ingredient lists.

Challenge: I'm not getting the support at home that I need to implement this new lifestyle.

It's difficult to make dietary changes when you're the only one in your household committed to doing so. This challenge is undeniable.

I'd suggest attending a support group. Many hospitals, clinics, and community centers have established groups of people who are making healthy changes to their diet, and there are also many online groups on Facebook and other websites as well. I create these for my own patients, and they report a huge increase in commitment when they come to these groups. In gatherings like these, we can share strategies for making healthy boundaries with our families/friends/coworkers around food. Another benefit to attending these groups is they strengthen another spoke on the lifestyle wheel, social connection. I love any strategy that combines two or more spokes of the lifestyle wheel, because when my patients intertwine these aspects of their lives and daily routines, their odds of success also increase exponentially.

Busting Common Food Myths

Finally, I want to look at two of the most common and prevalent myths around food. These contradict one another, and are at the center of many current disagreements about health and nutrition.

Myth 1: We need to eat meat and dairy to be healthy.

FALSE.

With the exception of vitamin B_{12}, which we'll discuss below, plant-based diets can provide all the required nutrients necessary for vibrant health. Regarding protein, we have twenty amino acids that are the building blocks to make protein. Nine of these amino acids are essential, meaning we can't make them or build them—we have to derive them from our foods. Historically, there were thought to be incomplete proteins that lacked one or more essential amino acids compared to the complete proteins found in animals. At the time, this was the basis for the belief that animal protein was superior to plant protein. However, these conclusions have since been proven false.[17] The bottom line is that eating a plant-based diet will in fact deliver sufficient protein and the essential amino acids needed without the baggage that animal protein provides, like cholesterol and saturated fat.

Vitamin B_{12} is an essential vitamin that we need in order to maintain our nervous system and the formation of red blood cells.[18] Like the nine amino acids above, we can't produce it ourselves and have to obtain vitamin B_{12} through the foods we eat. It's true that many animal sources contain vitamin B_{12}, but it's not produced by animals, it's produced by bacteria; for example, vitamin B_{12} used to be something we might have obtained by drinking well water, but due to our contemporary need to sanitize our drinking water by chlorinating it, that's no longer a source for us.[19] For those who do not consume animal sources, I do advise them to take a vitamin B_{12} supplement. However, there are no current dosage recommendations by any professional organization, and there have also been recent studies that suggest that high doses of vitamin B_{12} may be harmful, so I ask my patients to take the smallest dose available.[20] If you are concerned about your vitamin B$_{12}$ level, I recommend that you have your vitamin levels checked at least once every two years, if not every year, so you can make an informed decision with your doctor on the correct dosage for you. The only other possible vitamin supplement I may recommend to my patients is vitamin D; however, the larger conversation about vitamin D and any other vitamin deficiencies that may be affecting your health are really best discussed with your doctor, as they can order the recommended tests that will determine if vitamin supplements like vitamin D are indicated for you.

I believe animal sources in your diet should be minimal if included at all; in fact, I suggest if you are going to consume animal products, keeping these to only 10 percent of your total caloric intake. This is an educated guess, however; I do not have a clinical study that supports this advice. While I can cite several studies that reinforce the importance of a fiber-rich diet in improving disease outcomes, not one of them looked at a strictly plant-based diet specifically.[21] I personally believe that if they had added this aspect to the study, they might have seen even better outcomes, but this has not yet been proven, so again this is a subjective opinion. Know, however, that the foods I want you to consume the most are *indisputably beneficial* to you; fruits, vegetables, whole grains, legumes, nuts, and seeds are rich in fiber, plant protein, phytonutrients, vitamins, and minerals. If you choose to consume animal products (which have no fiber or phytonutrients and often include cholesterol and saturated fat), then I recommend that you choose lean meats, fish, and low-fat dairy options, and limit your intake of these overall. Eggs, if eaten, should be consumed sparingly.[22] Consider reducing how many eggs you have a week, and instead substitute with a food like oatmeal that has indisputable health benefits. When it comes to dairy, calorie for calorie, green leafy vegetables serve a more generous dose of calcium than dairy, with the added bonus of fiber and phytonutrients.[23]

I also want to note that although I conceded on the steak example earlier in this chapter, ultimately I do hope you will work to eliminate red meat from your diet completely, because the consumption of red meat has been linked to several poor outcomes, including cancer. I realize this change may not come all at once, so reducing meat intake for now is a step in the right direction. Remember, the changes we are implementing are lifelong. I don't want you to just stop eating red meat for six months; my hope is that you will give it up altogether, and for some people, tapering off is often the key to success when it comes to making a lifelong change.

Myth 2: Eating animal products of any kind is bad for your health.

ALSO FALSE.

So is this book pushing veganism? It is not. This book leans wholly on science and evidence. Vegans do not consume any animal sources, but they may (and often do) consume processed foods (foodstuffs). So being vegan is not necessarily in alignment with the research about what constitutes optimal nutrition.

Many individuals choose to be vegan for reasons beyond medical recommendations. They might be passionate advocates of animal rights or environmental issues. My focus here is solely on diet and its effects on disease outcomes. I will not discuss geopolitical reasons for eliminating animal-sourced foods. Although I love animals and am keenly aware of concerns related to the environment, this is not why I promote the consumption of a whole foods, plant-based diet to my patients. I recommend this fiber-rich diet because I'm a doctor, and that's what the evidence in peer-reviewed literature supports is the optimal diet for overall human health. It's also been my personal experience as a patient.

With that said, and as I noted previously, the majority of the studies I am quoting are *not* based on strictly plant-based diets; instead, they are primarily plant-based. The participants in these studies are often eating limited animal sources, like lean meats, fish, and low-fat dairy products, and getting to healthy outcomes. Certainly all health-care professionals agree that we need to reduce saturated fat and cholesterol in our diet to improve health outcomes. I think that the most effective way to do this—on a personal and societal level—is to emphasize what we need more of and not what we need less of. I want you to *increase* your fiber content. To do this, eat mostly plants. Trying to find and maintain the "perfect" diet is enough to make anyone crazy and stressed, which will not lead to healthy outcomes.

Food Is Life

A final note of encouragement about food: Remember that food is not only a basic building block of our physical existence, it's a part of our cultural, emotional, and even sometimes spiritual lives. Food is life, but it is also a rich source of connection, celebration, and joy. As you shift your mindset toward a more whole foods, plant-based diet, I encourage you to look for these moments of celebration and joy. Many of us have been taught to approach food as an enemy with whom we must do battle, or at the very least as a potential trap requiring our constant vigilance. Instead, try to approach this time of transition as an opportunity for cultivating a grounded, engaged, and loving relationship with your food. Its colors, smells, and textures are often delightful; try incorporating mindfulness into your food preparation, enjoying the sounds and smells coming from your stove, the music playing while you're cooking, and the presence of loved ones in the kitchen or at the table.

Keep It Simple Review

Remember, everyone has a different approach to improving their diet and nutrition, and this can be a gradual process. Every change, even if very small, is a step in the right direction.

Here is an easy way to remember the 1-2-3 of healthy eating:

1. Eat mostly plants (a wide, colorful variety).

2. Choose real food (no foodstuffs).

3. Reduce (or eliminate) animal sources.

Take Inventory

Taking a food inventory is similar to the personal self-assessment we did at the end of chapter 2, and the same principles apply. Knowing where you're at right now can help you make strategic changes in a new direction. To that end, take a look at your fridge and pantry. Notice the percentage of contents that you would you say is "real" food versus foodstuff. Remember not to self-scold as you do so; this is about information-gathering. I also encourage you to write down your food intake for a couple of weeks to get a better understanding of your habits and tastes (see the food diary template in appendix A for a helpful starting point). This knowledge can help you experiment and make adjustments that add to variety or address a specific issue with food.

Food Brainstorming

Make a list of all the healthy foods you'd like to bring into your life. Remembering the food pyramid we covered earlier, start with the fruits, vegetables, grains, legumes, nuts, and seeds you know you already enjoy. From there, see if you can add to each category, either things you may not eat regularly but like, or things you are open to trying. Leave out the things you know you don't like for now. For example, a friend of mine has disliked carrots since he was little, and the prospect of trying to find a way to add carrots to his plant-based plate was causing more stress than any health benefits of carrots could offer, especially given the alternatives. My point is, if you really don't like a particular healthy food choice, leave it off your list.

Plan It Out

Planning meals in advance has so many benefits: it helps you stick to a plan you feel good about, and it saves money and valuable time shopping and cooking. Researching recipes with some ingredients in common is also a fun way to introduce more variety into your diet and keeps meal times exciting.

As you write your plan, remember to include all the meals—breakfast, lunch, and dinner every day—and also plan for snacks midmorning or midafternoon as needed. Do your best to not skip meals. There are many wonderful resources for recipes, from cookbooks to multiple sites online. When evaluating any recipe, remember the 1-2-3 of healthy eating: eat mostly plants, choose real food, and reduce or eliminate animal sources.

Rebalance a Favorite Dish

Try adapting your favorite dish into something more plant-centered. For example, if you're ordering something at a restaurant, this might mean asking the waiter to double the veggies and leave out the buttered rolls and dairy-based sauce or dressing.

Here's another example: My husband comes from a loving Italian American family with roots in Brooklyn, and one of his favorite dishes growing up was orecchiette with sausage and broccoli rabe. It brings him straight back to joyful Sunday afternoons with his entire family eating together. When I make this dish for my husband today, I double the amount of broccoli rabe, opt for a whole grain pasta, and substitute the sausage with cannellini beans. This dramatically improves the nutritional value of the dish while compromising little taste or enjoyment. Try revisiting your loving roots and play around with old family recipes. How might you increase the plant power of something you already love?

4

The Importance of
Movement Every Day

An early-morning walk is a blessing for the whole day.
—Henry David Thoreau

When I think of all the years I lived with MS before I began making the changes that I teach in this book, one of the things that seems the most unsettling to me now is how little I moved.

In fact, I tried my best not to move.

That's because my balance was so poor that even the simple act of walking could lead to falling and injury. Ultimately, I chose to use a cane for assistance, and as a young physician, wife, and mother, this was very embarrassing for me. I didn't want my children, my husband, or my patients to see me with a cane, to view me as someone who was having so much difficulty just getting around. In the early days, I would try to hide my illness by forcing myself to go without a cane. I was supposed to be helping others, and I didn't want anyone to feel sorry for me or be distracted from their own issues by having to think about mine.

I now regret all that time and energy I put into hiding my condition, and I wonder if my readiness to change might have come sooner if I'd been willing to accept where I was, been honest with myself about it, and worked from there.

If you are suffering from a chronic illness and the very thought of physical activity is frightening to you, I can relate. Looking back, I sometimes wonder how I knew I was ready to start moving more, much less start an exercise routine, but after my blueberry aha moment and resulting diet change, I knew the next thing I needed to address was movement. Doing so was not easy, and outside of my husband I had almost no support. My doctors advised against it, as much of the medical thinking at the time was that people with MS should limit exercise, out of fear that doing so could actually exacerbate the disease.[1] This is not surprising when you consider that in my own case, my MS symptoms would actually worsen when I tried to exercise. For example, if I peddled on a stationary bike for even five minutes, I would begin to lose feeling in both legs. My initial reaction would be to stop, in fear of hurting myself.

For people with MS and other demyelinating diseases, worsening symptoms can occur when the body's temperature is elevated as in exercising, going in a sauna, or even being outside on a hot, sunny day; this is known as Uhthoff's syndrome or phenomenon.[2] What I didn't know then, but would soon figure out, was that by doing a little each day, and building on it over time, I could overcome this.

When I first started, my husband had to help me get on the bike every morning (when I placed my feet in the pedal straps I could not even feel them!). I was only able to complete a few minutes of pedaling before my body temperature would rise, Uhthoff's syndrome would kick in, and my MS symptoms would emerge. After my husband helped me off the bike, I had to sit for fifteen minutes drinking cool water as a shower of pins and needles continued through my body.

Early on, I was concerned that even this short regimen might be worsening my MS. It sure seemed that way. Over time, however, I noted less and less difficulty. Today, I run, hike, or walk every day, typically three miles in the morning. Twice a week, I work on strength conditioning—my regimen consists of push-ups, planks, squats, burpees, and dumbbells. I never could have imagined in those early days that I would make it to this level of fitness, but this willingness only came after I accepted where I was, and became willing to start from there, no matter how small.

I am now a firm believer in the importance of movement when it comes to achieving optimal health. However, I definitely understand the obstacles facing many of us when it comes to adding exercise and movement into our lives. For me, it strikes me as especially ironic that I am such a proponent of movement and exercise when I consider the fact that for much of my life, well before I had MS, this was not the case.

"I'm Not Athletic."

Growing up, no one I knew would have described me as an athlete. Those who knew me as a kid are shocked that running is now a part of my movement routine. That's because back then, I developed a near hatred for running, largely due to the fact that I was so slow compared to other kids. I remember in elementary school, when it came time for organized footraces, we were divided into two groups: the fast kids and the slow kids. I was always in the latter group, and my nervous hope was simply that I would not finish last.

Furthermore, coming from an immigrant family, formal exercise wasn't something that was important to us culturally. Going to the gym or pool was largely seen as a leisure activity, something we had neither the time nor money to do. I see now how experiences like this would affect my view of myself as someone who is not "athletic," and consequently influence my movement habits as I got older.

When I think back to my formative years, it's clear that societal messages and cultural views influenced my actions around movement and exercise. Just as we discussed in the last chapter on food, this messaging can affect our personal choices in whether we choose to exercise or not, but unlike food, the messages we get in these areas can be more subtle and harder to spot.

Let me explain. As young children, almost all of us moved and exercised. Of course, we didn't call it that—we called it playtime. We chased each other in games of tag, swung on the monkey bars, and jumped in a swimming pool whenever the chance presented itself. But for many of us, as we grew older, this playtime, and more importantly physical movement in general, fell by the wayside. Always the curious scientist, I wanted to know why this occurs for so many. Was it just a consequence of growing up? If so, why do some people continue with exercise and movement and others do not?

When I talk to my patients who haven't been regularly physically active in years, one of the most common themes I hear is that at some point in their lives they adopted the idea that exercise and movement are something best done by those who are "athletic," and that this was simply not how they would describe themselves. When I dug deeper, I found that those who were even just a little overweight often said that going to the gym felt more like an exercise in negative self-judgment and comparison than a means to improve their physical health.

If you are someone who doesn't have a regular exercise routine, I'd invite you to consider how societal and cultural messages may have affected your ideas about topics such as exercise and physical movement. If you've had personal experiences like I did growing up, or if you see those fitness models on television and immediately go into comparison and self-shaming, my hope is that by the end of this chapter you will feel differently about physical movement and exercise. To begin this shift, I'd like to dispel a popular yet mythical idea about exercise as a cure-all.

I recently had a patient referred to my practice, a sixty-one-year-old man whom I'll call Jim, who had just had a stent placement for a 90 percent blocked coronary artery. Jim had been living on the edge of a mortal cliff—in danger of having a massive heart attack at any moment that most certainly would have ended his life in a matter of minutes.

Yet you never would have guessed that by looking at him.

Here he sat in front of me, looking as slim and fit as the models we see in gym membership advertisements and bragging about his physical accomplishments. He said his friends joked he had the body of an Adonis, and his employees at the multimillion-dollar business he owned referred to him as Iron Man. When I reviewed his medical history, I learned that he had been an avid college athlete, breaking records at the Ivy League school he attended, and had continued this athleticism after college, running several marathons over the course of his life.

Do you want to know how he celebrated after those marathons he ran? With steak dinners, alcohol, and cigars. As I probed further, I found he also spent eighty to one hundred hours a week at the office in what was an incredibly high-stress environment, lived alone after a nasty divorce from a few years earlier, and hadn't talked to his adult kids in months. Does this surprise you? Not me. Sadly, I see cases like this all the time.

Distorted social norms falsely lull some of us into believing that high-level athleticism is the trump card when it comes to achieving optimal health. Loosely put, the idea seems to be, "If I can do all of these superathletic things and I look like the models in the ads, then my health must be great." So this messaging can not only lead to feelings of shame for people who run slower than others or have different body types, but can also mask serious health problems hidden behind a "healthy-looking" body, just like Jim's.

So often when we think of physical activity, we think of it in terms of improving how we look. We are bombarded with cultural images that tell us that health and beauty are dependent on small waists or huge muscles, but this is the skin-deep view of exercise that advertisers want us to see. The truth is that the positive effects of movement go far beyond appearances, as exercise improves our sleep, our mood, and our metabolism. These are just a few of the benefits you're likely to feel almost immediately. The long-term benefits include increased bone, brain, and heart health, all of which lead to significant increases in longevity and healthier, happier lives.

In the last chapter, we shifted the question away from counting calories for weight loss to focusing on the simple pleasure of eating a diverse array of colorful, whole plant foods. This shifts the emotional impact of these lifestyle changes away from grim drudgery and toward vitality and joy, and the same approach can be applied to exercise and movement. So rather than ask, "What exercises can I do to improve my appearance?" instead ask, "What fun physical activities can I start and stay consistent with in order to achieve optimal health, feel stronger, more energetic, and have a more positive outlook on life?"

Movement Is Medicine

Patients are often surprised when I say that movement really is medicine—and powerful medicine at that. I write prescriptions for it regularly, and I'll ask you to write your own prescription at the end of this chapter. But before we do so, let me make the scientific case for why movement is so important.

Physical activity reduces the risk of myriad chronic diseases, supports longevity, and improves quality of life. This is especially true for those who have been diagnosed with a chronic illness or are at risk for developing one. As is the case with every other spoke on the wheel, exercise cannot stand alone. You can't outrun a bad diet, and by the same token, you can't eat your way to the kind of bone, brain, and muscle strength you gain by engaging in regular physical activity. Let's take a look at the science and merits of physical activity in disease prevention and its value in longevity with a few facts that bring the data to life.

More than half a century ago, British scientists found that those with sedentary occupations such as the drivers of London's double-decker buses were likelier to die of a sudden massive heart attack compared to the city's more active professions such as postmen.[3] Scientists have also noted how over years, as more workers have transitioned from active jobs into sedentary office work or other jobs that kept them sitting for long stretches, heart disease has continued to rise at alarming rates. Researchers wondered if moving less meant higher risk of coronary artery disease (CAD). Recent evidence has shown sedentary behavior may be yet another risk factor for CAD, adding to the list that includes smoking, hypertension, and having high cholesterol.[4] Only about one in seven Americans smokes these days, and most of those who do wish they could quit and know it's bad for their health. Most likely, you'd consider it unhealthy to light up and puff away. But do you get that same sinking feeling about sitting at your desk for eight hours a day? Probably not—in fact, in many jobs you're expected to stay put and keep working!

Imagine you went to your doctor for an annual physical, and before leaving the room she handed you a one-word prescription: MOVE. It might seem peculiar, but she just offered a potent prescription, proven to reduce risk of the following:

- Heart disease

- Stroke

- Hypertension

- Type 2 diabetes

- Alzheimer's disease

- Obesity

- Postpartum depression

- Anxiety

- Depression

- Injury from falls

- Several types of cancer (bladder, breast, colon, endometrium, esophagus, kidney, stomach, and lung)

- Multiple sclerosis

- Attention deficit disorder

- Parkinson's disease

Plus:

- Decreased pain from osteoarthritis

- Improved cognition in dementia

Furthermore, we now have strong evidence that regular exercise is linked to improved quality and duration of sleep and reduced risk of depression and anxiety, all while optimizing executive function like organizational skills, planning, memorizing, processing, attention, academic performance, and improved overall quality of life. Adopting an active lifestyle means you will not only drastically cut your risk of developing a chronic disease, but you can also expect to be well-rested, mentally sharp, and happier! The simple yet powerful medicine of movement offers more benefits with lower risk of side effects than any drug available.

Of all the aspects of lifestyle medicine, diet and exercise are certainly the most familiar. We instinctively feel their connection to health and have likely heard about the benefits of doing both many times before. Yet despite this, trends of rising chronic disease and obesity continue. Why is this? In my view, the missing piece is making changes and sticking to them. Simple, but not always easy. How do we get these benefits when so much of our personal and professional lives seems engineered to keep us glued to our seats like those London bus drivers? How do we become more like mail carriers when we have demanding jobs, long commutes, and feel so tired by the end of the day that we fantasize about flopping onto the couch to unwind in front of the TV? And how do we do this in light of the societal messages that leave many of us more discouraged than energized, especially when we see all those images of how healthy bodies are "supposed" to look? Despite all of these legitimate barriers to keeping a regular exercise practice, I went from walking with a cane and shunning physical activity to running a marathon. I know that if I can do it, believe me, you can do it too.

Get Ready to Play

The first step to transforming your life through physical activity is less about your body and more about your mind. I'd like you to change your mindset away from thinking about movement as a chore or something you need to do to improve or maintain your physical appearance and begin to think about it like play.

In my first discussions with my patients, I often ask them to remember their favorite activities from the past, such as biking, dancing, or playing catch with a family member. In this way, we see if we can add some play-like activities to our movement routine. If swimming laps or running on a treadmill feels like unpleasant work, how about walking or hiking outdoors or learning to golf? With this shift in mindset, all of a sudden you get to choose from so many fun, playful activities that also happen to meet your movement goals, and this can help make whatever you do more sustainable and consistent as well.

On my Sunday walks or runs, I often see a large group of men in their forties playing soccer at the park. Those guys aren't getting together to meet their doctor's physical activity guidelines; they just enjoy soccer and want to play, play, play. In my eyes, however, they're also reducing their risk of heart disease, diabetes, and myriad other physical illnesses!

What I have also found is that when it comes to a mindset shift, this is a process that takes time and practice, trial and error, until you find activities that work for you. I know that some of you reading this have spent many years holding on to your current beliefs about physical activity and exercise. Commit to redirecting your thoughts until you get used to the idea that movement can be fun and that you can actually enjoy the benefits it brings.

Fun on Repeat

Do you remember falling in love with a certain song as a teenager or young adult? You would play it over and over, for hours at a time. When something is fun, we tend to get into a groove in the same way. So part of being ready to move is being open to experimenting until we find that activity we just can't get enough of. We also have to keep mixing it up as we go, so that we're always ready to discover new activities or commit to new goals. I have a friend who rediscovered her love of horses as an adult. Though she hadn't ridden in years, she started to take beginner classes. Being near these calm, powerful animals made her feel excited and empowered, and the extra activities of grooming and caring for the horses made it a real workout for her. I previously mentioned my friend who took up tennis at forty-three, and he's in better shape now at fifty than he was when he started. What I didn't tell you is that his coach, whom he has continued to play with a couple times a month since he started, is now seventy-five. My friend regularly tells me, "He runs around that court like a kid. It's an inspiration."

What fun, challenging, physical activities would you like to try? Line dancing, rock climbing, hiking, skating, bowling, and even shuffleboard are just a few examples of ways to begin moving while having fun too.

Physical Activity versus Exercise

So far in this chapter, I've been using both "physical activity" and "exercise" interchangeably. Let's get a little clearer on the difference:

- **Physical activity** is any movement that expends energy. Walking to your front lawn to pick up the newspaper or carrying the groceries in from the car would qualify as physical activity.

- **Exercise** is physical activity that is planned, structured, repetitive, and designed to improve or maintain physical fitness, performance, or health.

For our purposes, let's divide exercise further into two categories: aerobic exercise and strength training. Aerobic exercise is activity in which the body's large muscle groups move in a rhythmic manner for a period of time. Examples of aerobic exercises would be walking, running, or cycling, and it's one of the best ways to improve overall physical health. That being said, aerobic exercise won't get us the maximum benefit alone; for that, we need to add some strength training into our routine. While strength training is often associated with lifting weights, it certainly doesn't have to include those. Squats, push-ups, sit-ups, and the like are all examples of strength training exercises that don't involve any equipment other than your body.

When it comes to physical activity, the question I am always asked first is, How much do you need to move to achieve optimal health? While the specific answer varies from person to person, for the purposes of this book, it makes sense to stick to the simplest guidelines that are sure to benefit most everyone for health and healing, and those are outlined by the United States Department of Health and Human Services:

- 150 to 300 minutes of moderate-intensity aerobic activity or 75 minutes of vigorous aerobic activity per week (anything that gets your heart beating faster counts)

- And muscle-strengthening activity at least two days each week[5]

For aerobic exercise, the physical activities we described as play can go a long way toward meeting our needs here. Hiking, walking briskly, and dancing are all examples of that. The time allotment toward aerobic

INTENSITY OF EXERCISE	TALK TEST
Light	Can easily talk or sing Heart rate 63% or less of maximum
Moderate	Can talk but not sing Heart rate 64–76% of maximum
Vigorous	Difficulty talking Heart rate 77–100% of maximum

activity is directly connected to the level of intensity—light, moderate, or vigorous. The "talk test" is the simplest way to assign intensity. As your heart rate and oxygen needs go up, it gets harder to talk or sing.

By increasing intensity from moderate to vigorous, we can cut the time in half. In other words, from a lifestyle medicine perspective, you get the same health benefits from running at an eight-minute-mile pace for thirty minutes (vigorous) as you would from walking for an hour at a sixteen-minute-mile pace (moderate).

Strength training, on the other hand, isn't measured by time, but rather by sets and repetitions that target specific muscle groups. For most people, the physical activities we described in the section on play won't be enough to meet our strength training goals. Certainly there are times when they do, like when you help a friend move and your day is spent lifting and carrying boxes and furniture, but in general, this goal is best accomplished by doing exercises that strengthen the muscles in your arms, shoulders, chest, core, legs, and hips. This can be done with or without weights (sit-ups, push-ups, planks, and squats). For a good strength training routine, you'll want to do two to three sets of eight to ten repetitions of each exercise that works these muscle groups, and do this at least two times per week, but not on consecutive days, as it's important to give your muscles at least one day off in between to recover (I'll provide a sample script later in the chapter, when we dive into the details of strength training).

Jump Start: 150-Minute Deficit

I begin each week acknowledging I'm in debt. I owe my body at least 150 minutes of physical activity plus two strength training activities to give it what it needs and keep me at my best. I start at zero on Monday, even if I ran a marathon on Sunday. By starting this way, I set an expectation for myself. Each day, I chip away at this deficit and often find that by the end of week that I'm far in the black.

This can be made into a game where you challenge yourself to meet and surpass expectations. Of course, we are all starting at different places, so it's important to set goals that make sense. You might go back to your initial assessment from the Introduction as you're considering where to begin.

If you are sedentary with physical limitations, you might start with a five-minute walk each day, or as I did, with a one-minute ride on a stationary bike each day.

If you are minimally active, consider a step counter or adding an app on your phone that measures distance over time. Set a goal to increase your daily steps or time spent walking and gradually ramp up over time.

If movement is part of your daily life already (i.e., your job requires you to walk several miles each day), this might be the time to add strength training, adding one plank hold per day or five squats to start.

However you choose to begin, I encourage you to write down your goals in your journal. This way you can keep track of your progress and won't miss out on the sense of pride and accomplishment of doing this consistently over time. My patients often surprise themselves by looking back at their early fitness goals and seeing how far they've come.

An Rx to Move

As we make goals to sit less, move more, and gradually increase our structured aerobic and strengthening exercises, writing a prescription can be a powerful tool. I started doing this for my patients several years ago on the recommendation of the American Medical Association and the American College of Sports Medicine.[6] The Rx takes the form of the acronym FITT:

- Frequency

- Intensity

- Type (of exercise)

- Time (duration of activity)

I tailor each prescription to a patient's baseline fitness level, so here's an example of one I might write to meet the physical activity quota:

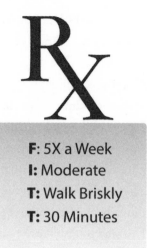

F: 5X a Week
I: Moderate
T: Walk Briskly
T: 30 Minutes

When I hand my patients an exercise prescription like this one, it feels tangible, legitimate, and serious. It serves as a concrete reminder that exercise is powerful medicine. On more than one occasion, I've had patients tell me that holding the signed prescription in their hand really changed how they perceived and valued the role of exercise in their overall health and well-being.

Walking: The Perfect Physical Activity

Walking is my favorite physical activity because everyone can do it, and you don't need to learn any special skills. You can easily adjust intensity and distance and set goals to build up your stamina over time. Walking at a moderate pace allows for talking, so I encourage walking with a companion (adding the social connection spoke of our medicine wheel while you're at it!).

I'm not alone in my love for prescribing walking as a form of exercise. Have you heard of an organization called Walk with a Doc (WWAD)?

It's the brainchild of my dear friend, cardiologist Dr. David Sabgir. Frustrated by the fact that few of his patients were meeting the minimal physical activity guidelines, he made a desperate offer to one of his most entrenched patients: Will you walk if I meet you at the park and walk with you? Not only did this patient say yes, but so did another hundred patients. Since that moment back in 2005, Dr. Sabgir has never looked back—and WWAD has grown to several hundred chapters.

As a proud walk leader for the organization, I have personally witnessed the value of walking together. In this community, we share conversation, wellness strategies, and recipes and develop lasting friendships with like-minded individuals—all of which serves our overall lifestyle medicine prescription. I highly recommend joining your local chapter of WWAD—they are all over the country and have international chapters as well.

Speaking of suitable companions, did you know that dog owners are more physically active, calmer, and more social?[7] Even petting your dog has been linked to reduced blood pressure and heart rate.[8] Adopting a dog is a big responsibility, but they are great motivators to meeting your physical activity needs.

Recently, at the behest of my kids, our family visited an animal shelter under the condition that we were just going to visit and there was *no way* we were going to adopt a dog. While there, the young man showing us around made a comment from which I could not walk away. He mentioned a sweet dog named Barney who was beloved by everyone there, but they felt was unadoptable as he was both old and had an autoimmune disease. Now I had to meet him—we had so much in common! Within seconds, I knew he was ours. He engulfed my children with his loving demeanor, and I found myself driving this elder statesman home with us. He is the best walking buddy I could ask for.

Strength Training

When it comes to the strength training part of the weekly recommendation, many people struggle—even those who are meeting the minimum goal of 150 minutes of physical activity. I urge you to make time for this crucial supplement to your exercise routine. Not only does strength training offer us the benefit of strong bones, muscles, tendons, and ligaments, but when we are strong we are at lower risk of injury, more easily maintain a healthy weight, and enjoy overall improved quality of life.

You should engage in strength training exercises twice a week, with ideally a twenty-four to forty-eight-hour rest period in between sessions. There are any number of online and print resources that show simple beginning exercises using your own body weight for resistance. You might also choose to supplement this routine with resistance bands or light hand weights, but this is totally optional.

When writing a strength training prescription, I include the force or weight being used, and the number of repetitions and sets. Repetitions are the number of times the weight is lifted in each set—typically, you want to repeat the lift until you reach muscle fatigue. This may take eight to twelve reps per set. If you find the lift much too easy or difficult, then adjust.

Here's an example of what a strength training script might look like:

1. Push-ups or knee push-ups, 10–12 reps

2. Plank, hold for 1 minute.

3. Squats, 15 reps

4. Bridge, 15 reps

Repeat circuit above three times.

Though most of us can increase our aerobic activity with few issues, fewer people are comfortable with strength training on their own. There's good reason for that, since it's important to avoid injury and assure good form. I often suggest that my patients go to a physical therapist or exercise professional, or take group classes at a gym or studio, to learn or tune up resistance exercises. But physical fitness does not have to be expensive. You don't need to join a fancy gym or purchase pricey equipment. I largely advise using your own body weight for resistance exercises at least to start, and walking for aerobic exercise.

Yoga as Strength Training

When it comes to strength training, most people think immediately of weight lifting; but yoga can be a great way to add some resistance work to your weekly routine. One of the things I love about yoga is that it has variations for almost any age group, and it is something that many who enjoy it continue to practice well into their advanced years. Even if you've never tried it, chances are good that you've already heard of yoga; in the last few decades it's become one of the most popular forms of movement in the United States.

While yoga is thousands of years old and has its roots in the spirituality of India, over the years it has traveled and adapted to different countries and cultures, and in the United States it is primarily an exercise-based practice, though there are certainly yoga studios and traditions in the United States that still emphasize spirituality as well if that is appealing to you.

In addition to enhancing muscle strength and flexibility, yoga has the added benefit of engaging the breath and centering the mind into a stress-reducing meditative state, and classes with others can also enhance your social connections (two more spokes on the lifestyle medicine wheel!). There are a wide variety of health benefits to yoga, including lowered stress level, relief from anxiety and depression, relief from some forms of chronic pain, and improved sleep (another lifestyle medicine spoke!).[9]

In yoga, as in other kinds of strength training, the weight you are lifting is your own body weight. As you build muscle, you may need to increase the time spent in a pose or up the number of repetitions to get the maximum benefit, but this is also true of weight training.

Yoga can be intimidating for some people because the prevailing media image of an average yoga practitioner implies that you have to be young, athletic, and superflexible (and be able to practice on the tops of

mountains, empty pristine beaches, or dramatic volcanic rock forma-
tions). None of these things are true. Yoga can be for any body.

There are many, many different types and traditions of yoga to
choose from; some kinds focus on slow, meditative poses (like yin
yoga), some on intense physical exertion (like Ashtanga, vinyasa, and
power yoga), some on spirituality (kundalini yoga), and so on. There's
even aerial yoga, where you perform various yoga poses while hanging
from a special hammock bolted to the ceiling! The fact is that yoga can
and has been successfully adapted to accommodate a variety of physical
needs and differences.

If you are new to yoga and want to give it a try, start by visiting the
yoga studios in your area. Major cities will have many of them, but even
a growing number of smaller cities are starting to see at least one or two
yoga studios nowadays. The YMCA and other gyms often offer yoga
classes as well. I suggest speaking with some of the certified instructors
at these places and explaining to them that you want to try yoga as a
means of strength training, and they can advise you if the type of yoga
they offer is a good fit. Many studios offer introductory rates for first-
time students—some may even be donation-based—and almost all will
be able to provide basic supplies such as yoga mats and blankets if you
don't have your own. As with any new practice, don't be afraid to start
out slow and easy and build from there. Your goal is to begin a strength
training practice that you can stick with and build on for years to come.

Keep Going with Consistency and Connection

Before we go further, I want to emphasize the importance of consistency. We all know that exercise is good for us (and hopefully now you
know *just* how great it is!). And yet many of us struggle to stick with our
goals. Of course we lose out on all the benefits of movement if we stop
doing it altogether.

This can be a challenge. In my case, moving was uncomfortable,
and initially it seemed to make things worse instead of better. Some
of my patients struggle with feeling embarrassed or discouraged by

their starting point. I encourage you once again to ease up on any self-judgments. It's very difficult to make progress of any kind when we can't be honest with ourselves about where we are and accept that's just what *is* right now. Our current burden of illness, upset, pain, or struggle does not define who we are.

I used to think I could predict which patients would do well and which would not within the first visit. After many years, I've learned that I really cannot know what any one person's potential might be. Why? Because potential is inherently unknowable, a story we tell after the fact when we see how things have played out. When it comes to transforming their health and well-being, I've had patients surprise me in many ways. I will say this: the only way you can know your own potential is to try every day. The patients who choose to be consistent, who ask questions, who don't miss appointments, and who do the homework open up new doors of untapped potential. I've seen them overcome chronic illnesses and go on to live happier, healthier lives. How? Day by day, moment by moment. One choice at a time. And, most importantly, *by being consistent.*

In this section, I'm going to give you a few ways to keep things consistent, interesting, and on track. These are only a few of the infinite possibilities, so I encourage you to experiment and see what works for you.

Plan It Out

Just as we discussed with planning your meals, you are much likelier to complete your physical activity requirement and strength training routine if you plan it out. Just as you set time aside to clean out your pantry and prep ingredients in the last chapter, you can also optimize your schedule to achieve your exercise goals in the same way. Begin by considering what your schedule looks like right now. It may seem at first that there is no flexibility or opportunity to add a new activity, but by shifting your mind a little bit, you may find more moments for movement than you previously thought possible. For example, ten, twenty, or even thirty minutes out of a lunch break can be a great time to take a brisk walk (which has the added effect of reenergizing you for the afternoon), or you may find that by waking up just ten minutes earlier than usual, you've created some time you can spend riding a stationary bike, going for a quick jog, or doing a few sun salutations (a popular yoga sequence). Once you've determined where and how long you can add movement to your week, you can write yourself a prescription and set concrete, realistic goals, such as "I will walk for ten minutes on my lunch break every day for the next four weeks," or "Mondays, Wednesdays, and Fridays I will go for a thirty-minute evening walk; Tuesdays and Thursdays I will do strength training at home; and Saturdays I have a tennis date with my friend Charlotte." Here are some other tips and suggestions:

- Schedule a regular walk or workout session with a reliable friend for accountability—boost each other whenever needed, and problem solve to get past obstacles. Cold weather? Move your walk to an indoor mall—or suit up and enjoy the crisp, refreshing air.

- Consider trying to do movement first thing in the morning when you're likelier to be full of energy, as opposed to trying to exercise after work when you may be fatigued and/or overwhelmed by responsibilities at home like cooking or taking care of family.

- You might find it helpful to put on your walking shoes first thing in the morning, or keep a set of sneakers in your office, so you can transition seamlessly into your exercise time no matter when it might be.

- Sign up for a yoga, water aerobics, or other group class— prepaying for classes sometimes makes us more consistent, because we like to get our money's worth. Classes also have the added benefit of providing opportunities for social connection.

- Schedule family time outdoors doing something that requires walking, hiking, bike riding, etc. For example, trips to botanical gardens, parks, and museums all often require quite a bit of walking. Make a family game out of trying to visit every park in your city, county, or even state.

- Reinvent your personal image with affirmations such as "I always take the stairs," "I am strong and capable," or "I'm an active, outdoorsy person." Or come up with a family motto, like "This family makes time to have fun outside on Saturdays."

- If you find yourself resistant to the word *exercise*, relabel your physical activity as something more interesting to you. For example, your daily walk may be a hunt for great photographs to take or a search for natural objects to incorporate into an art project.

Exercise Snacking

The more you move, the better—even if it's a little. I have a friend who's at risk for blood clots when she flies in an airplane, so she sets an alarm to get up and walk down the aisles every half hour. She recently realized she can do this at home or work as well, and every time her bell goes off she jumps up for a quick stretch of her legs.

Doing a few jumping jacks, stretching, or adding steps to your normal routine can make a difference. I like to call these bite-size physical activities "exercise snacking." Like grabbing an apple and a few almonds midafternoon, they can boost your energy and your metabolism and help you achieve your health goals at the same time. They also chip away at your 150 minutes of physical activity for the week. If you take the parking spot farthest away from the front door of your office, it may take you three additional minutes to walk to your car every day. That means you've just added thirty minutes of aerobic exercise by the end of the work week, leaving you just 120 minutes to go. With this simple step you've met 10 percent of your weekly goal!

Here are a few other examples from my own routine:

- Every Monday afternoon I have a set scheduled teleconference with colleagues that typically runs an hour. I used to take the calls from my office, sitting at my desk. A few months ago, I started taking these calls while walking at a comfortable pace on my treadmill. I often forget I'm walking! This gives me a full sixty minutes of moderate aerobic activity to add to my weekly total.

- My office is about 2.5 miles from my home. It's a very short drive, but I often choose to bike or walk there, turning a five-minute drive into a thirty- to sixty-minute heart-healthy commute. Active commuting has been shown to reduce cardiovascular risk by up to 11 percent.[10] Is it possible to introduce some element of active commuting into your life? Could you get off at an earlier subway or bus stop and add some steps? Maybe walk the kids to school rather than drive them? One good rule of thumb is that if it takes five minutes or less to drive there, consider walking.

- Last year, I found myself binge-watching a popular television series, so I moved from my living room couch to my stationary bike. I was entertained and met my daily dose of movement!

Now it's your turn. What are three ways you can ditch the sitting and become more active?

Attractive Activities

Whenever someone tells me that they're having trouble sticking with a goal, I ask them if their options attract or repel them. Funny as it sounds, when it comes to physical activity, we should check in about whether or not we even like something, because more often than not if something about it repels us, even just a little bit, we're far less likely to do it.

For instance, I love the feeling of being outside in almost all weather. I like to pay attention to birds, plants, and the change of seasons, to feel the wind in my hair. For these reasons, I'm attracted to running and walking in the little nature preserve by my house. If I tried to confine my running and walking to a treadmill, I would be far less likely to stick with it. Of course, some people are the opposite—they would much rather watch TV or listen to music while on the treadmill. The trick is to find out how you can make your physical activity more attractive to you.

Here's another example that shows how the inverse of this can work against you. I bought a brand of shoes that, after a couple of runs, I just didn't like as much as the ones I normally wore. Even after the break-in period, they weren't as comfortable as I wanted, but I thought I "should" wear them because I had paid for them, it was too late to return them, and they were technically good shoes. Within a few days my runs were getting shorter, and I was feeling less motivated to run and likelier to find excuses not to do it. Then I realized it was all because of the shoes! I promptly gave them away, and it was a big relief to get another pair of shoes that I loved to put on. My running and motivation returned immediately. My point here is to review all the details that go into the physical activity you choose, especially if you are having trouble getting and staying on track. Making even a few small changes can set you up for success rather than failure.

Keep It Simple Review

- Aim for at least 150 minutes of physical activity plus 2 sessions of strength activity per week.

- Incorporate play into your routine. Exercise should be fun and freeing, not a chore.

- Remember, consistency is key. If you don't meet your goals for the week, get back on track as soon as you can.

Recover and Retune

Creating a fitness feedback loop can help you make continuous progress. To do this, write down your ideal fitness situation for this week or month (this could be your prescription, for example). Second, write down your current experience, as objectively as possible. Finally, articulate the difference between those two things. For example, *My body works best when I do yoga twice a week and walk to work every day. Right now, I run out of time to walk in the morning. I'm managing to do yoga once a week, and only sometimes twice.* Now focus on the difference, without judgment: *I'm going to prep for the mornings the night before so that the decision to walk is already made in the morning. My friend Peter goes to yoga—I'll try making a set plan to go to a class together.* In this way, you can consciously evaluate your progress and retune your goals.

1 Percent Better

Fitness practitioner Mark Fisher shares a powerful motivating strategy, which is to think of ways that you can get 1 percent better today. This approach always seems doable, and I return to it again and again. If I've taken 100 steps, 101 is certainly no big deal—but doing this day after day means that before long I'll be taking 1,000 and then 10,000 steps. The compound interest that makes investors rich can help you improve your fitness in dramatic ways.

A friend shared with me the advice to floss just one tooth. The thinking behind this is that the most challenging thing about keeping a healthy habit is overcoming the inertia of not doing it and just getting started. If we tell ourselves we are just going to floss one tooth, it feels like less of a chore. Of course, once the floss is out and you've begun, it's no problem to quickly finish off every tooth. Applying this to movement and exercise, you might tell yourself that you'll just walk for fifteen minutes, and then add "just one more minute" every day/

week. You may find that you're soon walking for twenty, thirty, or forty minutes at a time!

Shoes in the Pantry

You know how much I advocate walking as the best means of starting and sustaining a physical activity routine. Here's a simple life hack I love to help you meet your goals in this area. Author and researcher Brené Brown says that she keeps a Polaroid picture of her walking shoes taped to the inside door of her pantry. She realized that when she was bored, restless, or stuck on a page of writing, she often found herself opening that pantry looking for a snack. Seeing the shoes reminded her that getting outside for a walk almost always helped her solve problems, elevate her mood, and reset her ability to work better than any snack could. This is a perfect example of how the spokes on the lifestyle medicine wheel can work together: diet, exercise, and a peaceful walk can help you reduce stress and reset, just as it does for Brené.

A Slow Climb

Part of making sustainable change is building incrementally. One patient of mine became obsessed with her step counter as a way to measure her daily progress. Pretty soon, however, she ran into a problem: she would push herself one day and see a big spike in her steps, which was great, but then noticed the next few days would be much lower than her monthly average. This yo-yo effect wasn't leading to overall gains month to month. So instead of going too fast, she made a simple goal: take more steps than my lowest count for the month, every day. Over time, this meant that she was always increasing her steps slightly, and able to be more consistent about her progress.

Your Prescription

Go ahead and write yourself two prescriptions in your journal—one for aerobic activity and one for strength training. Make it something you know you can do at first, and faithfully take this "medicine" for two weeks. At that time, reevaluate just as a doctor would, and adjust the dosage in terms of time, intensity, or number of sets. Put reminders in your calendar to do this every two to three weeks, as this is a great way to build and sustain fitness goals over time.

Here are some examples of prescriptions you may write for yourself:

Aerobic activity:

- 5x a week, light, walk around the office during lunch, 10 minutes

- 3x a week, moderate, walk in the neighborhood, 20 minutes

- 1x a week, moderate to rigorous, dance class, 90 minutes

- 1x a week, rigorous, hiking with Jeremy, 2 hours

Strength training:

- 2x a week, yoga DVD, 30 minutes

- 2x a week, push-ups, 10 reps x 5 sets

- 2x a week, squats, 15 reps x 3 sets

A Crazy Goal

I've already mentioned that my first "crazy" goal was inspired by my brother's suggestion that I run a marathon. This goal reoriented my thinking and changed the way I perceived myself—not as a patient defined by my illness but as a person and physician empowered to take on big challenges and prevail. In 2015, I set a goal of walking 2,015 miles in one year (a little more than five miles per day) to commemorate the major milestone of living with MS for twenty years. Back when I was diagnosed with MS in 1995, the doctor told me at my bedside that I would be in a wheelchair in twenty years. When I look back on 2015, it was not easy. I walked five miles no matter what the weather or how I felt. There were days I did not want to get out of bed, but I did it, never missing a day. On October 11, 2015, the twentieth anniversary of my hospitalization, I celebrated by walking twenty miles accompanied by family and friends for the final five miles. This year, for my twenty-fifth MS anniversary, I plan on walking twenty-five miles.

Sometimes I'll ask my patients to envision what might feel like an impossible physical goal. It could be anything from climbing a mountain to swimming a certain number of miles in a year. I find that particularly for patients with chronic illnesses, just shifting to thinking big in this way starts to loosen up our preconceived ideas about what we're capable of and opens up new pathways to healing. Take some time and journal about what might seem like a crazy goal for you. Put it aside and look at it again in a week or two and see how you feel.

Living Better with Mindful Stress Management

True silence is the rest of the mind, and is to the spirit what sleep is to the body, nourishment and refreshment.
—William Penn

In 2007, four years after starting my intensive lifestyle changes, I went through a dark and difficult period. I had accepted a new position that allowed me to be closer to home, but the stress associated with the job was overwhelming. About a year after taking this job, I ended up in the hospital for two weeks. I will share the full details of how and why this happened later in the book, but for now I want to mention this time in my life because of the profound impact it had on me in terms of the importance of stress management.

You see, even though I was eating and exercising well, sleeping through the night, etc., my lifestyle plan wasn't in check when it came to stress. Looking back, I see now that I was acting as if I could somehow overcome the stress in my life by focusing on other aspects of the lifestyle medicine wheel.

As a side note, I can tell you that after helping countless patients over the past several years adopt the lifestyle changes I am describing, the attitude I had around stress management no longer surprises me. In other words, I have often noticed that some patients will skimp on one spoke of the lifestyle medicine wheel, either consciously or unconsciously, because they think that area doesn't really apply to them, or that they can handle it, or that they will make it up in other areas, etc.

Unfortunately, I have also seen this backfire on patients time and time again, as neglecting one area of the lifestyle medicine wheel can keep them from experiencing the full benefits they desire. Ironically, it's often the area we think we don't need any help with that actually requires the most help. That was certainly the case for me when it came to stress management, and I share this with you in hopes that you can avoid this trap.

Returning to my life in 2007, and because of what I was going through at this time, a dear friend shared with me a copy of Viktor Frankl's book *Man's Search for Meaning*, in which the author chronicles his horrific experiences as a prisoner in a concentration camp during World War II. It may seem like a strange gift to give a struggling person, since the book details the unimaginable brutality Frankl endured during his imprisonment. He recounts his fear, anger, starvation, exposure to extreme cold, and relentless uncertainty about his own fate, as well as the loss of his father, mother, brother, and wife, each of whom was murdered in the camp. In this atmosphere of total devastation and inhumanity, Frankl discovered something incredible. Survival, he writes, is dependent on finding meaning in life. Purpose and meaning guide us through the most difficult of times. One of my favorite quotes from the book that sums this up is as follows:

> *Everything can be taken from a man but one thing: the last of the human freedoms—to choose one's attitude in any given set of circumstances, to choose one's own way. . . . When we are no longer able to change a situation, we are challenged to change ourselves.*[1]

This was the gift my friend gave me, the guidance that would allow me to accept and even embrace my pain. If we can't change the circumstances of our lives, we must become willing to change ourselves. Suffering occurs when we stay focused on fighting circumstances beyond our control, or when we *resist what is*, rather than accepting and changing what we can, even if that is just our perception of it. By resisting reality, we not only waste precious time and resources, we also resist the opportunity to begin the kind of life transformation we crave and deserve. I described this kind of resistance in the last chapter when I discussed having to face my own physical limitations before I could move forward with an exercise plan. I needed to start in reality, with what I *could do*, not what I *wished I could do*.

Peace becomes available to us the moment we accept our circumstances, regardless of their nature. Religious and spiritual traditions across the globe carry this universal message as well. With this outlook, we find a master key to dealing with the inevitable stress each of us encounters in life. Through acceptance, we come back into the present reality—the only place we can take meaningful action—and we no longer allow stress and suffering to curtail our potential.

As we look at the stress spoke of the lifestyle medicine wheel, we'll discover how to halt and reverse the damaging effects of stress on our physical and mental health. It's important to remember that stress itself can never be eliminated from human experience. Indeed, we wouldn't want it to be, since it plays an important role in our ability to perform and achieve. But when we shift our perspective, as in so many areas of our health and wellness, we gain insight. There's a lot we can do in a general sense to work with the stress in our lives, and there are many specific tools I will share with you in this chapter.

Before we begin, I ask that you be open to the idea of changing yourself rather than changing your circumstances. Subtle as it may seem, this internal change is a heroic feat, one that can lead to profound individual transformation, not to mention optimal health.

What Happens When We're Stressed?

In my opinion, too many of my colleagues in medicine underemphasize the role of stress in health. Just as medical schools and hospitals largely ignore the overwhelming evidence about the benefits of a plant-based diet, stress and the simple techniques used to manage it are often relegated to a side corner, maybe feeling more like the domain of self-help than science. There is plenty of hard science, however, that demonstrates the dangers of being overstressed, as well as the profound benefits of practices like mindfulness and meditation. I know from personal experience, as well as from the dramatic life transformations I see in my patients, that the effects of chronic stress cannot be denied when it comes to our health, especially for those of us dealing with chronic illness, which brings its own added stressors.

Let's briefly look at the mechanics of stress and how too much of it can be a very bad thing.

We can think of stress as something that evolved to keep us safe, alive, and thriving. When a predator jumps from the bushes, or when it feels like the social group around you might get angry and force you out, your brain and body go into high alert, making all resources available to minimize whatever threat you are facing—real or perceived. If we were to make an analogy between our body and a computer, we could say that the brain is like a neural "motherboard" that accepts external input through our senses and processes an internal response, identifying what's dangerous and what's desirable at a mostly subconscious level. So while your brain is largely in charge of this process, you don't have to *think* about ducking when a ball comes flying at your head. The stress response happens in a matter of nanoseconds. The brain sends and receives messages through the central nervous system, which travels through nerves to all corners of your body and in turn communicates with the cardiovascular, immune, and endocrine systems.

This system works best when it can rest and recover between spikes of heavy traffic. When humans experience constant stress (or chronic stress)—even at a low level—the overwhelmed body and brain start to suffer. High stress can impact everything from blood vessels (leaving us more susceptible to heart attack and stroke) to the endocrine system (gumming up the hormone responses that control everything from mood to proper digestion). In this way, chronic stress can lead to chronic disease.

Researchers have linked many chronic diseases to high stress levels, most prominently heart disease, the number one cause of death.[2] This is not surprising in our current stressed-out world. Similarly, metabolic disorders like diabetes and obesity are more prevalent in individuals who are of lower socioeconomic status, a particularly highly stressed segment of our population. Consider the stress of someone whose daily concerns might include surviving in a high crime area, poor environmental conditions, and limited job opportunities.[3]

Stress's damaging effects can be reversible in the short term, but they can become permanent when endured over extended periods of time. When we experience acute stress, cortisol is released from the adrenal gland. This hormone suppresses function in the hippocampus, resulting in impairment of memory. Continued relentless stress can actually shrink the nerve cells in this important part of the brain. Believe it or not, even this brain shrinkage can be reversible in the short term; but if stress continues over years, we effectively *kill* our neurons. We see evidence of this in MRI studies of patients living with chronic stress, such as those diagnosed with post-traumatic stress disorder or major depression.[4]

Stress puts pressure on the immune system as well, which calls up armies of white blood cells to prepare for battle in the event of acute stress. This can help fight off infection in the short term, but when it happens constantly over time, it can wear down the effectiveness of the immune system, resulting in autoimmune disorders, allergies, and decreased cellular immunity.[5] When chronic stress impairs immunity on a cellular level, it might lead to a severer cold or recurrent upper respiratory infections. In other words, being sick while being stressed means feeling worse for longer.

My patients often relay to me that after a year or two of lifestyle change, they notice a big difference, saying things like, "This year I got through the entire winter without bronchitis, sinusitis, or a cold." These statements don't surprise me anymore, and I will share stress-busting lifestyle changes in this chapter that will fortify your immune system.

Although it is important to administer yearly flu shots, it is a missed opportunity when we neglect counseling patients on the importance of optimizing their lifestyle to strengthen the body's immune response. Imagine if we all made these changes in addition to getting our yearly flu shots. The flu might not stand a chance.

Finding Your Sweet Spot

While unhealthy levels of stress are clearly detrimental in a variety of ways, it's important to point out that having some stress does play a positive role in our ability to perform and achieve. We need enough stress to stimulate our brain, muscles, and even our gene "switches" so that we stay healthy and responsive to our environment. Too much stress, on the other hand, leads to poor physical and mental performance in the short term and to long-term degradation of our social, emotional, and physical well-being.

One of the tricky things in dealing with stress is that no two people define a "stressful" event or situation in the same way. Think of two individuals who are required to jump from an airplane wearing a parachute. One of them interprets this as a miraculous opportunity to fly, while the other feels sure he's plunging to his death. This is an exaggerated example, but the point is that people can view and respond differently to the same exact situation.

While we can't pinpoint what is going to be stressful or not stressful to every person in every situation, the key is to learn about your own responses to stress and what you can do to better manage those. Normally in lifestyle medicine we're trying to address the cause of a problem rather than the symptoms, but in the case of stress it's a little different. While causes of stress can and should be examined, we're very often looking more closely at the effect of something that's stressful and how we perceive stress in general. We want to figure out how to alter our perception of stress, as well as our brain and body responses to it, so that we can maintain a healthier equilibrium.

In order to do this, each of us has to locate our own "sweet spot" of stress—how much is enough for us, but not too much. The figure below shows a stress response curve based on an idea first developed by psychologists Robert M. Yerkes and John D. Dodson back in 1908.[6] The theory is that performance improves with increasing stress, but only up to a certain point. After that, there's a dramatic decline in function.

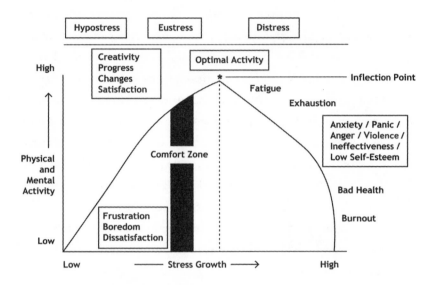

Notice on both sides of the curve that physical and mental activity is low. When a kid is bored at school, for example, with nothing to challenge them, they might be in this state. Too little stress (*hypostress*) leaves us dissatisfied and unproductive. But as stress levels climb, we enter a period of creativity and growth referred to as *eustress*, or what I call the sweet spot. Here we are challenging ourselves to achieve, produce, grow, and promote progress. This kind of stress serves our overall well-being as we find ourselves purposeful and contributing in a meaningful fashion. But once we push beyond our threshold, we rapidly descend into *distress*. This is what you probably think of when you think of stress—the physical and mental sensations of exhaustion, anxiety, suffering, and/or anger that can be overwhelming.

This stage of distress also leads to bad outcomes in decision-making, increased risk-taking, and poor overall health. So how much stress is good? How much is acceptable before we tip the scales and crash and burn? The answer is different for any two of us, so the goal is to find out what is best for you. We can build the skills to recognize our personal stress sweet spot, and we can learn to employ coping mechanisms that improve our limitations when it comes to stress response.

Here's an example from my own life: When I'm traveling for work, I know that I will be carrying a heavier stress load. Navigating unfamiliar places, speaking in front of large groups, and even having slight changes to my regular patterns of sleep, nutrition, exercise, and meditation all contribute to higher stress levels in a negative way. However, I also find these trips invigorating—I'm learning, sharing, and doing what I love. During a recent conference, I realized that I was beginning to feel tired and irritable. I've learned to tune in to these particular warning signs; I could feel that I was slipping over and beyond my stress sweet spot. One night toward the end of the trip, I had to reconsider whether I would attend an important dinner event. Going to the dinner would mean losing extra sleep, which I knew could set me back even further, so I politely told the host I would not be attending. It's not always fun to make that decision and lose out on an experience, but when I put it in the context of my overall health and wellness, the decision was a no-brainer.

This is a simple example, but my point is that stress can be both positive and negative, and where the sweet spot is can be different for everyone. Some people seem to be able to perform under massive pressure, while others have a low threshold for stress when dealing with everyday tasks. In either case, it's important to find and pay attention to your own sweet spot and learn how to return to balance again and again. If chronic stress is leading to difficulty sleeping, overeating/undereating, or constant fatigue, you've overdone it and are now in treacherous territory. When this happens—and we've all been there—we have to be willing to make an adjustment. The rest of this chapter will provide a basic framework to address the general underlying stress that can wear down our health, as well as powerful ways to target specific stressful moments so that you can successfully return to your sweet spot again and again.

Our level of vulnerability and resiliency to stress is influenced by multiple factors, including our genes, environmental factors (childhood abuse, conflict-ridden households, difficult socioeconomic conditions), and behavioral factors (social instability, mental illness). Each of these factors interacts with the others and changes over the course of our lives. Our experiences and life events mold the "motherboard" of our brain as we go, a process referred to as *neuroplasticity*.[7] The good news about neuroplasticity is that we can change our brain and recondition our stress responses. Just as eating mostly plants renews our gut microbiome and regulates our weight and blood sugar and exercise improves our cardiovascular health and switches on powerful genes to protect our well-being, we can optimize the brain and nervous system to stay in balance and increase our resilience. Even those who have had significant trauma or damaging experiences in the past can recover and transform their stress response. With preventive measures, including lifestyle medicine interventions in diet, exercise, and social integration, we can make transformational change, fortifying our brain and body to better sustain future stressful events.

Where to Start

Everyone knows in general what it feels like to be overly stressed, but to effectively deal with stress, we need to get specific. When I evaluate patients, I break stress symptoms down into three areas: physiological, behavioral, and psychological. *Physiological* signs may include headaches, loss or gain in appetite, fatigue, diarrhea, erratic speech, weight loss or gain, and increased blood pressure and heart rate. *Behavioral* symptoms include emotional outbursts, irritability, excessive alcohol use, isolation, inattentiveness, and sleep disorders. Finally, *psychological* signs commonly include anxiety, depression, and suicidal thoughts. Stress may not be the only factor contributing to these symptoms, but by treating stress in some specific ways, many patients experience significant alleviation of many of their symptoms.

One of the biggest barriers to the treatment of stress that I see in my patients is an unwillingness to engage with stress management *before* these symptoms get out of hand. As with nutrition and exercise, societal messaging is part of the problem. Often we are told to simply "muscle through it," "toughen up," or "get over it" when it comes to feelings of stress. Most of us internalize this type of self-talk without realizing it, and we give ourselves a hard time when we're suffering as a result.

If you take some time to listen to the voice in your head, you will likely find that you speak to yourself in ways you would never speak to anyone else. For instance, if you saw your best friend struggling, or you saw a crying child in need of assistance, I'm willing to bet your first response wouldn't be to tell them they're being ridiculous or that they should push aside whatever they're feeling and toughen up. Yet this is exactly how so many of us speak to ourselves in moments of stress. While this type of negative self-talk may seem effective in some cases, it is ultimately a shortsighted solution that carries long-term risks when it comes to your health, not to mention it creates a lot of mental suffering in the process.

Like all the other changes I am advocating in this book, the first step is to shift your mindset. There is no better example of the need to do this than with stress, which almost always begins—and can end—in your mind. Returning to the theme at the beginning of this chapter: the foundational approach to dealing effectively with stress is being willing to change what you can while accepting what you can't.

Chronic Stress

At certain times in our lives, stress can be more like a general feeling rather than something related to a specific event or situation. In these instances, stress can often be the result of a combination of things, such as dealing with your own chronic illness, taking care of a busy family, or navigating a difficult situation at work. When dealing with situations like these that are largely beyond our control, attending to the other spokes of the lifestyle medicine wheel can help support stress reduction. Here's how:

Adopt a healthy diet. We've already explored how food affects our physical health and chronic disease progression in profound ways—but does food really influence our mental health? The emerging scientific evidence says this loud and clear: *YES.* In a 2014 review of more than a dozen studies, authors concluded that a diet rich in fruits, vegetables, whole grains, and fish was associated with reduced depression risk.[8] An Australian study showed that a group of young adults who ate more fruits and vegetables and reduced processed foods, saturated fats, and refined sugars were able to significantly reduce their symptoms of depression, anxiety, and stress.[9]

Engage in daily exercise. Physical activity can literally rewire the brain, improving mood and reducing psychological stress via the complex neurobiological framework of the central nervous system, including the release of favorable endorphins and chemical mediators.[10] In layman's terms, the evidence is overwhelming that adding more exercise to your day benefits your brain and moves you closer to that optimal level of stress. The excitement of playing a pickup basketball game or the challenge of a new hike can turn on the positive stress circuitry.

Check in on sleep. We'll be talking about sleep in more depth later in the book, but it's important to note that stress, and particularly anxiety and depression, often interfere with healthy sleep cycles. This can include everything from insomnia to extreme fatigue that keeps you in bed all day. Effective sleep hygiene allows the body and brain to reset and repair the cells and neurons that can be overtaxed by stress.

Practice mindfulness and meditation. While there are many relaxation techniques and activities such as massage, taking a warm bath, or gentle stretching, I think of mindfulness and meditation as two of the most powerful tools available to alleviate stress. These approaches have been proven to be effective in study after study, yet they're still not widely embraced by most Americans.[11] They're simple, free, and can be done almost anywhere at almost any time.

Mindfulness is the practice of bringing awareness to your current experience, from the sensations inside your body to what you perceive with your five senses in your environment. It is the willingness to be with what *is*, right now, in the present moment, while letting go of judgment. So many of us are constantly thinking about the future or the past, and the practice of mindfulness is about focusing our mind on what is happening in the now.

Meditation refers to many practices that increase mindfulness, from sitting quietly with our eyes closed, focused on our breathing, to a walking meditation in which you focus on your environment and body sensations. Meditation often helps us distinguish between our thoughts and feelings, on one hand, and our *awareness* of these thoughts and feelings, on the other. You might think of your awareness as the sky, and your thoughts and feelings (stressful or pleasant) as clouds or weather systems that pass through this awareness. A regular meditation practice helps us to notice the difference between the two, allowing us to become observers of our stressful thoughts and feelings so that they are less likely to feel like a permanent storm. I often repeat the mantra "This too will pass" when I'm experiencing something that seems heavy and unbearable. This too will pass. Nothing is permanent.

Meditation and mindfulness practices support reduced stress responses in the nervous system, and they can boost physical health as well by decreasing blood pressure and heart rate and improving respiratory function. Remember, each spoke of the lifestyle medicine wheel bolsters the effectiveness of the other spokes, and meditation and mindfulness practices are just another example of this. If you are new to mindfulness and meditation, there are some exercises at the end of the chapter to help you get started.

Reduce your substance intake. While almost everyone knows that reaching for a cigarette isn't a good response to a stressful situation, having a glass of wine or other alcoholic beverage to "take the edge off" a stressful day is not only widely accepted, it's often encouraged. But this is a short-term strategy with long-term consequences. We'll discuss drinking later in the book, but for now suffice it to say that our goal in dealing with stress is to do so *without* the use of outside substances.

Stay connected and get support. Stress and loneliness can create a vicious cycle. The worse you feel, the less likely you might be to engage with the people you care about, which will in turn make you feel worse. Surrounding yourself with supportive friends, family, and loved ones and sharing with them how you are feeling will go a long way to decreasing the negative health impacts of stress. In addition, others are able to offer perspectives that we maybe haven't considered.

One caveat here: Depending on your situation, some family members and friends may not be a good resource when it comes to dealing with stress. For instance, if there's someone in your life who is prone to seeing the negative in most situations, they're likely not someone you should reach out to for support during moments of stress. They may be a great friend and an ally in other areas, but knowing who is best to seek out when you are experiencing stress can often be the key to feeling better.

In addition, some life situations require more structured support groups. These can be especially helpful for those with chronic illnesses, alcohol or drug addiction, issues of grief and loss, or for those seeking specific lifestyle changes. Finally, don't hesitate to seek help from a mental health professional. If you are overwhelmed, having difficulty coping with a challenge, or having suicidal thoughts, seek immediate medical care. There is always a solution to every problem.

Acute Stress

When stress is tied to a specific situation or event, the importance of a shift in mindset can't be overstated. Whenever you feel yourself getting stressed, ask yourself, *Do I have influence over this situation or event? Could I make a decision or act in a way that could help alleviate this immediate stressor?* If there is nothing you can do, it's important to *accept* that.

Here's a simple example. A friend of mine had planned a surprise party for his wife's birthday at a nearby lake, with fancy caterers, boat rentals, and a local band. The week of the party, the weather forecast turned ominous; they might get rained out. In the final days leading up to the party, my friend constantly checked the weather forecast, lamented about how the rain would ruin his plans, and grew more and more upset. Finally, the day before the party, he accepted the fact that it would either rain or it wouldn't, and there was absolutely nothing he could do about it. Now free from the burden of worry, he was able to adjust his plans. He bought ponchos for everyone and moved the band's setup to under the park pavilion. Yes, it did end up raining that day, and while the boating plans were canceled, many danced under the pavilion instead, and a good time was had by everyone—especially his wife, who loved all of it.

My friend's experience is certainly a minor one in the big picture of life, but I like it because it underscores the importance of recognizing what you can and cannot change. When we learn to recognize and let go of things that are beyond our control, we can then spare ourselves the mental anguish and adverse biological consequences. This frees us to make choices about what we *do* have influence on.

Consider my own example about declining an invitation to an important dinner. Because I have learned through experience that I need to put self-care first, I declined something that I really wanted to do because I knew the better answer for me was to rest and get a good night's sleep. This was an instance when I accepted the situation that I was exhausted as it was and made a decision to choose a different path, avoiding more stress in the process.

Here are some additional tips for shifting your mindset when dealing with stress around specific situations and events:

Take the next smallest step. When my child is overwhelmed by a school project, I ask her what the smallest step would be that would move her toward her goal of completion. Breaking a big problem down in this way minimizes the debilitating pressure of getting the whole thing done at once, and doing one next action offers a sense of completion that can fuel progress toward the bigger goal.

Don't sweat the small stuff. Very often I find that stress is fueled by relatively small things, and we often lose sight of our biggest priorities in the midst of it. We have an unexplored dumping ground in our head of things we "should" be doing—everything from dusting the coffee table to applying for graduate school. We can't do everything at once, and in fact we won't be able to do everything we want to do, period. We only have a finite amount of time on this earth, and if we don't take time regularly to sort through our to-dos and link them to specific goals that are important to us, we can quickly get overwhelmed and over-stressed. Who cares if your coffee table is dusty? Live your life to its greatest potential today. Prioritize and don't overextend.

Time management flows from clear priorities. Did you ever notice how much you get done at work in the week before you leave for vacation? Because you know you'll be unreachable

(I hope!), you have a specific set of goals and a specific timeline. Everything else you have to let go.

Give yourself permission to say no. Saying yes when you really mean no is a surefire way to create stress in your life. Take a look at those situations where you agree to do something out of a sense of obligation rather than a genuine desire to do so. If a friend asks you to have coffee but you know you want to go running instead, it's perfectly fine to say you have other plans. (In this instance, you could even blame me and say, "I'm going running—doctor's orders!")

Now, I realize that there will always be situations when we must take action even when we don't want to, but these are typically fewer and farther between than we realize. Allowing yourself to say no can be a life-saving skill. I used to worry that folks would be disappointed if I didn't attend their event or respond to every email or social media post. But I realized that in the end none of these were all that important, and I was ultimately serving my patients and my community better by tending to my health and well-being.

Renegotiate your commitments. This was a powerful lesson for me. As a good student and a perfectionist, I've spent a lot of time in life being hard on myself for not living up to expectations—mine or someone else's. Then I embraced the idea that everyone is allowed to renegotiate their commitments on an ongoing basis, with themselves and others. This allows me to work with setbacks and stay focused without the heaps of self-judgment I used to rely on for motivation. Think of it this way: it might feel terrible and stressful if you can't pay your phone bill on time. Maybe you had an emergency or some other unexpected expense. You might tell yourself that you're failing as a provider, and you might be angry with yourself or think it's not fair. The phone company is almost always willing to renegotiate. Give them a call and set up a payment plan or ask for a onetime extension. This process can apply broadly in your life. Missed your exercise goal this week? Renegotiate! Morning routine creating stress for everyone? Renegotiate as a family and try something new. Keep yourself honest, but don't punish yourself. That's counterproductive.

One last thing. Whether or not you can change your situation directly, and whether or not you're beginning to have a handle on making the profound lifestyle changes in this book, I want to remind you of the single most powerful way to change your relationship to stress: *be kind to yourself*. We all make mistakes. We all fall short of our goals at times. When this happens, remember that you are a human being. Pain, suffering, and difficulty are all part of what it is to live a human life—as are joy, connection, and love. You can take personal responsibility for any mistake you make without sinking into shame and blame, and then let it go. Acceptance is key, and self-forgiveness is powerful medicine. Lighten your load. Your body and mind will thank you.

Keep It Simple Review

- Find your stress sweet spot and practice rebalancing over and over again as new situations arise.

- Support yourself by practicing mindfulness and meditation.

- Pay attention to the other spokes of the lifestyle medicine wheel: eating, exercise, sleep, and connection.

- When you have control over a situation, take small steps to minimize stress. When you don't have control, remember that you *always* get to choose your reaction and your perspective, no matter what.

• Be kind to yourself—especially when you fall short of your goals.

Gratitude List

Gratitude is one of life's amazing gifts, and there is even evidence to suggest it has real physical effects on the body. A psychology experiment conducted in 2003, for example, found that when one group of people was asked to write down the things they were grateful for and another group was asked to write down things that annoyed them or even that they felt neutral about, members of the gratitude group exercised more regularly, reported fewer physical complaints, and had a more optimistic outlook on life in general compared to those in the negatively focused group.[12]

Of course, you likely don't need a study to tell you that expressing gratitude makes you feel good inside. Still, there are many days when feeling grateful may be hard to do—especially if you are suffering from a chronic illness. However, by incorporating a regular gratitude practice into your day, you can improve your mindset in general and perhaps lower your stress level in the process. One easy, fast, and deeply rewarding practice is to make a simple gratitude list, either in the morning or at the end of each day—or both!

For this exercise, write down at least three things that you are grateful for today. These can be little things, such as the cup of coffee you are drinking as you write, or big things, like the people you love the most or a community you are glad to be a part of. Don't worry if you don't have some magnificent list of grand moments to record; the purpose is to find something you feel grateful for, be it big or small. On a bad day, it's fine if all you can come up with are seemingly tiny things, like "I'm grateful for the pillow supporting my back right now," "I'm grateful for the color of this wall because I picked it out," or "I'm grateful for this pen—it writes well."

Here's an example from my own gratitude list:

> *I am grateful for this tasty cup of coffee.*
>
> *I am grateful for my husband and children—they make my life so fulfilling.*
>
> *I am grateful for the difference that lifestyle medicine has made in my life and in the lives of countless others.*

If you're stumped, here are a few prompts to get you going: Any good weather today? Did you eat something that tasted good? Were you able to take a short break today? Did you see or talk to a friend? Is there something you love in your home you can be thankful for? Do you have any pets? Did you hear a good song today?

Once you've made your list, reread it slowly and carefully, bringing the thoughts and feelings of gratitude into your body and mind. Just as stressful thoughts can produce negative emotions, practicing gratitude can help you feel positive emotions.

You can keep this list in a special gratitude journal, add it to your regular journal practice, or even jot it down on sticky notes and then leave them around the house to find later.

My point here is that nothing is too small or too big to be included in your gratitude list! Try to do this daily for at least two weeks, as many people who do so happily continue the practice after that because it feels so good.

Mindful Walking

For this exercise, go outside and take a thirty-minute walk at a comfortable pace. Don't worry about whether you're getting a good workout or not—just try to keep your attention focused on your surroundings:

notice the sights, the sounds, the scents, and even the taste of the air. As you walk, it's likely your mind will begin to wander to what's happening later that day or what happened yesterday. When you notice that, simply bring your attention back to the present. If it's helpful, remind yourself that you can think about all of those things later, after your walk, but for the next few minutes you'll be paying attention to your surroundings. If you are like me, you may have to bring your attention back to the present moment several times during your walk, and that's perfectly OK.

The benefits of mindful walking are twofold. One, you give your mind a break from all the habitual thinking, which can help lower your feelings of stress. Two, when you engage in mindful walking even at a very comfortable pace, you encourage the release of favorable chemical mediators in your brain. This makes you feel good. Imagine if you did this walk every day; the flow of positive neurotransmitters would serve you on a daily basis!

Meditation

Meditation often seems intimidating to many of my patients who haven't tried it. Popular misconceptions about meditation include things like you have to do it for lengthy periods of time, assume difficult postures, or go to special spaces such as remote temples to do it "correctly." There is also a common misconception that meditation involves somehow controlling your thoughts. In my experience with meditation, none of these things are true.

You can benefit from a meditation that is only a minute or two long, it can be done seated in a chair, walking, or even running, and the only special space I recommend is a place you can be alone and undisturbed for a few minutes. Perhaps most importantly, meditation is about allowing your thoughts to simply be there, observing them rather than attaching to them. Meditation is simply an invitation to rest your mental muscle. With that in mind, try a seated meditation, for as little as five minutes.

Quick Steps to Meditation

1. To begin, find a place where you can be undisturbed for the next five to ten minutes. I recommend sitting in a chair or on a cushion on the floor—anywhere that allows you to be comfortable yet alert (so you don't fall asleep). Set a timer for five minutes. If you use your smartphone's timer, put it in airplane mode so you won't be interrupted.

2. Close your eyes and bring your attention to your breath. Notice your inhale and exhale, and feel your chest and stomach expand and contract. Pay attention to the feeling in your nose and mouth as the air goes back and forth through them. Your mind will likely begin to wander. This is normal. When you notice this has happened, simply allow the thought to be there and bring your attention back to your breath.

3. When the timer goes off, you're done! How'd it go? If five minutes was too long, then start with just two minutes. Eventually, try to work up to twenty minutes of meditation, three times per week.

Many people find that they are calmer in the days and moments between their set meditation times, and as a result they continue meditating regularly. If you are having trouble doing this alone, you can look for meditation groups in your area. There are many different types, religious and secular alike. Another option is to consider downloading suitable apps on your phone/device to support this new practice.

Establishing Good Sleeping Habits

Sleep is the golden chain that
binds health and our bodies together.
—Thomas Dekker

At one point in my life, I considered myself a hopeless insomniac. A combination of factors including high stress, poor nutrition, lack of exercise, and dealing with the symptoms and treatment plan of my MS left me unable to get a night of restful sleep for months, and then years. Slowly but surely I became addicted to hypnotic drugs like Ambien, and also depended on the occasional use of benzodiazepines like Ativan. These medications kept me in bed and unconscious for at least a few hours in a row, but they never gave me the physical and psychological benefits of real sleep. I felt sure that I would never be free from these drugs, would never get a full night of restful sleep, and would never overcome the debilitating effects of insomnia I experienced night and day.

Thankfully, I was wrong.

I am pleased to say that I now sleep very well the vast majority of nights, and I no longer need any medications to help me do so. While I hope you aren't experiencing the level of difficulty with sleep that I was, I do know that healthy sleep can be a challenge for anyone—especially those living with chronic conditions. Overcoming insomnia was incredibly difficult for me, especially in the backdrop of dealing with my MS. I'll share with you how I did it in this chapter, and I'll give you the tools you'll need to enjoy the benefits of healthful sleep yourself.

For some of you reading this, sleep may not feel like quite as com-pelling a topic or as essential to your health and well-being as some of the other areas covered in this book. You may believe sleep is wasted time, and that most people can, and do, get along fine with limited hours in bed. I assure you that nothing could be further from the truth. Sleep is one of the most underappreciated contributors to our overall health, cognitive abilities, and emotional stability. Chronic lack of sleep is an important indicator of serious health problems as varied as diabe-tes and heart disease, not to mention the fact that the risk of death from accidents of all kinds is far higher for those with a sleep deficit.[1]

In terms of the transformation you are undertaking through the principles in this book, you may have already begun to make some basic tweaks to your diet and exercise routines and bolstered your stress man-agement. Very often in my practice, I see people make changes in these areas first, and then ease up when it comes to the other spokes in the lifestyle medicine wheel. Why? Partly I think it's because most people who come to my practice are desperate for relief, and once their symp-toms ease even a little bit, they don't see a need to invest further time and energy in the long-term and difficult process of habit change. I have to remind them, in order to reap the greatest benefits of lifestyle change we must tend to all spokes in unison.

Here's an example: I commonly see diabetics who want to focus solely on diet and exercise and are surprised when I spend a good bit of time on the topic of sleep. In fact, a 2006 study concluded that sleep duration and quality were significant predictors of how well blood sugars were man-aged in type 2 diabetics.[2] A diabetic's bedtime may be just as important as their dinnertime—healthier eating *and* healthier sleep make more of a difference together than either could on its own.

So I'm going to urge you to incorporate each and every spoke into your transformation! You deserve it. By taking an honest look at the state of the other spokes on the wheel—how they are showing up in your life right now—you are giving yourself the best chance to feel better, conquer your chronic conditions, and dramatically improve your chances for a longer, healthier, and happier life.

What Makes for a Good Night's Sleep?

We all have to do it, and without it we wouldn't survive. You may be under the false impression that your body and mind just "turn off" at night, but that couldn't be further from the truth. It has actually taken quite a lot of scientific research to understand what's going on when we sleep, with new discoveries being made all the time. We are only now learning more about the ways that sleep affects our physical and mental health and our ability to function while awake.

You probably know that there are several "stages" of sleep, during which we experience different critical biological processes. Every night, we travel through each of these important periods, and we must spend adequate time in every stage in order to maintain wellness and feel rested in the morning.

Let's look at the journey of sleep we take every night and how the four stages fit into a healthy regenerative cycle. We have three stages of non-rapid eye movement (NREM) sleep, followed by one stage of rapid eye movement (REM) sleep. It takes about an hour and a half to go through all four stages, and a good night's sleep consists of moving through this complete cycle several times.

Here's what happens in one of these cycles:

NREM1: Slipping into sleep. Your brain waves begin to slow as you ease into the first relaxing stage of sleep. You are entering a very light sleep from which you can be easily awakened. Your eyes move slowly, muscles relax, and your heart rate and breathing slow down.

NREM2: Light sleep. There is a notable drop in your body temperature, heart rate, and blood pressure. Your eye movements cease and your brain waves slow way down, with occasional bursts of rapid waves.

NREM3: Deeper sleep. Your brain waves slow down even further. Now that you are in deep sleep, it's more difficult to rouse you. In this stage, much healing and regeneration occurs, including the repair of tissue, new cell growth, and the buildup of your immune system, among other things. If you don't spend adequate time in this stage, you will not feel well rested in the morning.

REM: Rapid eye movement sleep. About ninety minutes after falling asleep, you reach REM sleep. In this stage, you dream. Your eyes move rapidly beneath closed eyelids and your heart rate and blood pressure may rise, yet your muscles are temporarily paralyzed to protect you from acting out your dreams. This stage is important in learning, processing, and sorting information.[3]

Research indicates that we get the greatest health benefits in NREM3 and REM sleep. If we don't get enough sleep during the course of the night, we miss out on the regenerative and protective processes of these stages, thus setting ourselves up for dysregulation and disease.

Dangers of Disordered Sleep

Whether you have worked night shifts for years, struggle with occasional sleepless nights, or just decide to stay up another hour to finish a few things you want to do, losing sleep leads to profound health-related complications. If you avoid going to sleep because you think it's wasted time, you couldn't be more mistaken. Whatever work you do in the extra hours you stay awake will be slower and less productive, and it will come at the cost of your overall health. The cognitive loss you experience in sleep deficit is similar to having a blood alcohol concentration over the legal limit for driving.[4]

Despite the very real dangers of not getting enough sleep, however, our contemporary culture seems to encourage it. We are conditioned to be proud of not "needing" more than a few hours of sleep; we're told that this makes us hard workers, dedicated to our professions, or admirably unwilling to miss a single moment of our lives. We may repeat phrases like, "I'll sleep when I'm dead," or "Sleep is for the weak." An entire energy drink industry exists in intimate relationship to these false ideas about sleep and profits from keeping people up when they should be resting. The fact is that sleep is a fundamental human necessity, not a weakness, and sleep deprivation is not a sign of our dedication—it's a sign that we are overworked, overstressed, and damaging our health. I want us to stop celebrating people who sacrifice sleep, as sleep deprivation puts everyone at risk.

Insomnia is the most common sleep disorder reported by Americans and characterized by chronic difficulty falling asleep and/or staying asleep. Many factors may contribute to this, including stress, physical pain, depression, drugs, alcohol, and even some medications. Of course, we all on occasion experience trouble sleeping—that's normal. We call it insomnia when this issue goes on for three months or more. This condition can be treated and must be brought to the attention of a physician. Please do not delay seeking care from a health-care professional if you are experiencing ongoing sleep deprivation. The overview of sleep in this chapter will help you have a meaningful conversation with your doctor to get the best possible treatment plan.

In addition to insomnia, the other most common sleep issue I see in clinical practice is obstructive sleep apnea (OSA). Sleep apnea is a category of conditions related to irregular breathing during sleep. OSA is often related to obesity, as increased fat deposits around the tongue and throat restrict airflow, resulting in lack of oxygen and awakening from sleep. Many patients may not be aware that anything is wrong, and often the first clue comes from their sleep partner, who reports loud snoring with periodic frightening episodes when the individual appears to stop breathing. OSA may be present in almost half of those with a

BMI greater than 30. This is sobering, since the most recent obesity rate reported by the CDC is 42.4 percent.[5] This equates to many millions of Americans suffering from OSA. This condition is treatable and manageable, but the diagnosis needs to be made to prevent complications like heart disease and increased risk of motor vehicle accidents.[6] If you snore and/or experience daytime drowsiness, please bring this to the attention of your doctor for an appropriate evaluation.

Beyond these leading sleep disorders, I encounter patients dealing with restless legs syndrome, narcolepsy, sleepwalking, bed-wetting, nightmares, and more—all of which can complicate effective sleep hygiene. Whenever a patient is having trouble sleeping, it is important to take a detailed history and complete a thorough physical exam to fully understand what is contributing to this disruption.

In a recent case, a patient presented to me with what he described as inexplicable alertness and nervousness over six months, which was interfering with his sleep. In working with him further, I made a diagnosis of hyperthyroidism. Once we treated his overactive thyroid, his sleep cycle normalized. In another case, a patient was sleeping nine to ten hours, which is more than normal. Her blood work revealed she was suffering from iron deficiency anemia from uterine fibroids. Once her fibroids were managed by her gynecologist and iron stores were replenished, she reverted to a healthy regenerative sleep cycle. I share these examples to dissuade you from ignoring any sleeping problems you may be experiencing, as so many people do for years, and tell your doctor about them instead.

For all of us, it's not just the quantity of sleep that is important, but the quality of sleep too. That is, you might stay in bed for seven or eight hours a night without ever fully going through all four sleep stages. Inadequate or poor-quality sleep has been linked to several chronic diseases including heart disease, type 2 diabetes, stroke, obesity, and depression.[7]

There is even evidence that poor sleep habits like those practiced by irregular shift workers could contribute to cancer risk.[8] In a study published in 2013, investigators concluded that female night shift workers were at a 30 percent increased risk of breast cancer.[9] This might be due to the disruption of normal circadian rhythm (another name for our internal biological clock). Being in a light-filled environment at night suppresses the release of the chemical melatonin. Melatonin helps us feel sleepy and fall asleep naturally. When this cycle gets disrupted long term, it can be hard to get a good night's sleep.[10] That's why turning off *all* the lights in your bedroom may be one of the simplest and most important things you can do to improve the quality of your sleep.

Sleep disorders are indeed a global challenge, with Americans experiencing more trouble sleeping than other cultures. An international survey conducted more than a decade ago showed that 56 percent of people surveyed in the United States reported sleep problems, compared to 31 percent in western Europe and 23 percent in Japan.[11] Over half of Americans aren't sleeping well, and even if they know the health and safety dangers, very few folks ask for help from their doctors. When they do, physicians most commonly treat the sleep complaint with a prescription. Sound familiar? By now you know that there is often a better way than the prescription pad to address the root causes of chronic conditions through simple, profound lifestyle practices that elevate virtually every measure of health and well-being.

Getting Started on Your Journey to Better Sleep

We spend around one-third of our lives sleeping. If you live to be seventy-nine, that means you will be snoozing for a little more than twenty-six years! So how do you optimize all this sleep? There are some things you can do, using the principles of lifestyle medicine.

When I was ready to make a plan to improve my sleep hygiene, I really had no idea whether I could be successful at it. And things did get worse before they got better. If you've been using sleep aids to stay in bed and unconscious other substances such as alcohol, opiates, or cannabis for this purpose, this may also be the case for you. I urge you once again to be honest with yourself and to have faith that you can improve your overall health by learning how to sleep well without the use of these substances.

In my own case, the first step was to track all sleep habits. This increased my awareness about so much of what was affecting my sleep: diet, exercise, substance usage, light exposure, even the temperature of my bedroom. For example, I realized that the wine I was drinking with dinner at that time was playing a role in my insomnia, as was occasional ice cream or other sweets in the evening; these things may have felt good in the moment, but it was only temporary. In the long run they were interrupting my sleep cycle and affecting my health! In addition, I'd been keeping the television on in my bedroom as I fell asleep when my husband was away on call. Not only did my sleep improve when I removed the TV from the bedroom due to its light, but I also stopped watching the evening news in the family room before coming to bed because I discovered that it often upset me and kept me awake.

Armed with a strong sense of my sleep patterns and habits, the next phase of my sleep journey was to make a sleep plan. I purchased a physical calendar just for this purpose, and plotted out regular decreases in my sleep medication. (*Note: If you are coming off sleep aids, it is critical that this step be made in consultation with your doctor.*) This helped me anticipate difficulties and make a plan to overcome them. For example, I knew that for three to five days after a dosage drop, I might not sleep almost at all, which would make being productive almost impossible. These days were tough, and I was tempted to up the dosage again so I could resume sleeping the "easy" way. At the same time, I knew that was not what was best for my long-term health, and so I stayed the course. These were the days that I actually felt worse before I felt better.

I also wanted to make a checklist of supportive sleep habits in that same calendar, such as turning off or putting away technical devices two hours before bed, taking warm showers, praying and gratitude journaling (like the Gratitude List exercise in chapter 5), listening to soft music, doing deep breathing exercises, and even playing guided sleep meditations.

Having those resources all in one place made it easy to find them when I was in a panic at 3 a.m. and afraid I might never sleep again.

It also helped me to remember that the other spokes of the lifestyle medicine wheel could aid my sleep recovery journey. Eating healthy, plant-based foods meant I wasn't trying to digest a heavy meal with animal protein, high fat, and sugar as I slept. Exercising regularly meant that my muscles were tired and ready to rest. Stress management helped me practice breathing techniques and calm the anxiety that could often keep me awake all night. Becoming aware of substances I was consuming helped me choose to avoid caffeine after my initial cup in the morning, and not rely on a glass or two of wine to make me feel sleepy at night.

The last step was to consciously plan a fixed sleep structure. I had a set bedtime (9 p.m.) and a set wake-up time (5 a.m.), and I stuck to it as much as possible—even on the weekends (I know—but trust me, it's important to be consistent). I chose these times because they work best for me; I love the early morning hours when I feel most alert and alive. You may need to make small adjustments and find what works best for you.

Eventually, all of these small changes resulted in a complete 180 in my sleep pattern. Nowadays, I love sleep! I look forward to the time each day when I can wind down, pray, express my gratitude, and close my eyes peacefully, knowing that I am helping my entire being rejuvenate and be its best and most refreshed the next morning. By integrating these sleep skills into your own life (and it's a commitment!), you'll reap the same dividends of waking joyful, rested, and replenished.

Three Keys to Sleep Hygiene

The National Sleep Foundation defines *sleep hygiene* as a variety of different practices and habits that are necessary to have good nighttime sleep quality and full daytime alertness.[12] Note that this definition calls good sleep a *practice*. Just like meditation, exercise, etc., you're never going to be "perfect" at sleeping, and you'll want to keep fine-tuning your goals and strategies. Remember: your aim is to make changes that are sustainable for the rest of your life, and that means building practices rather than attaining specific goals. Effective sleep hygiene means addressing and optimizing both our environment and behaviors related to bedtime and sleep, which will give us many benefits in the long run:

1. Fall asleep effectively and consistently.

2. Stay asleep for an appropriate length of time.

3. Maintain a high quality of sleep each night and over time.

These are the three keys of good sleep hygiene, and of course they all overlap with one another. Many of the things that improve the quality of your sleep, for example, will also help you fall asleep more consistently. Breaking them down in this way allows us to target specific habits and practices to focus on each aspect of healthy sleep.

Falling Asleep

The physiology of sleep is complex and influenced by many factors, but it is largely driven by a hormone called melatonin, which is produced by the pineal gland in the brain. Sleep is managed by a light switch in the brain. It starts when the light sources in our environment are put out. These could be natural, like the sun setting, or mechanical, such as turning off the television or a bedside lamp. In the darkness, retinal ganglion cells in the back of our eyes communicate with the pineal gland in the brain via a neuronal highway, stimulating the release of melatonin, which makes us feel drowsy and ready for bed.[13]

We know that much of the difficulty we experience falling asleep can be tied to problems in this system. Most of us stay glued to our technology well after sunset, and screens emit enough light to inhibit the melatonin response, which can throw off the body's internal clock. This is an even bigger issue for shift workers who work nights and sleep during the day.

There are a number of things you can do to optimize your sleep experience:

- Your ideal sleep space should have a comfortable bed, pillow, and bedding. It should also be cool, dark, and quiet.

  Cool: Your bedroom should be slightly chilled, somewhere between sixty and sixty-seven degrees. This temperature supports the physiology of optimal sleep. As our body temperature goes down, it triggers sleep.

  Dark: Since light inhibits melatonin production, we want the room to be void of any light sources. I would recommend investing in blackout curtains/shades or a sleep mask. If you can, keep all light-emitting electronic devices out of the bedroom at night (this includes your TV and your smartphone).

  Quiet: Try to keep your bedroom as silent as possible. If you need to keep your phone close by, put it in airplane mode so you aren't disturbed by its vibrations or noises. And if street noise or other sounds are keeping you up, playing white noise from an app or running a fan would be good options.

- Most sleep experts recommend keeping the bedroom reserved for only sleeping and sex. That is, don't work, read, eat, or watch television in bed—especially if you are trying to change your sleep habits for the better.

- Reduce light exposure as the evening progresses. Use dimmers or turn the brightest light sources off in your living space during evening hours. Discontinue use of computers, phones, etc., at least an hour before bed. You may want to increase this to two hours if you are still having trouble falling asleep.

- Decide on one or two relaxing rituals around bedtime—for example, taking a warm shower or bath, or practicing ten to fifteen minutes of meditation. This last one will also help you reflect on and process any negative emotions or anxieties that might otherwise keep you up at night.

Staying Asleep

Many people who can fall asleep regularly might have difficulty staying asleep. Regular waking for any reason compromises a healthy sleep cycle. As a consequence, you may not adequately reach the stages of sleep where most of the health benefits occur.

The Sleep Council recommends that adults eighteen to sixty-five sleep seven to nine hours per night on a regular basis to promote optimal health. (For those over sixty-five, that number drops to seven to eight hours per night.)[14] I usually advise eight hours to my patients, and they regularly hear my motto: Sleep eight and you'll feel great!

Here are a few strategies for maintaining uninterrupted sleep:

Minimize late-night trips to the bathroom. Particularly as we get older, or with certain medical conditions, we may wake one or more times in the night to go to the bathroom. Cut down on this need by avoiding eating or drinking two hours before bedtime and emptying your bladder right before you climb into bed.

Don't drink alcohol before bed (or, better, don't drink at all). The relationship between alcohol and sleep can be confusing, since drinking in the evening can make us feel sleepy and might even make us fall asleep faster. But alcohol decreases the length and intensity of REM sleep (the regenerative fourth sleep stage) for the first half of the night, and then as the alcohol is metabolized, it wakes you up more often. We'll talk more about alcohol in the next chapter, but my strong advice is to not drink regularly or excessively for a variety of reasons, one of which being that it interferes with your ability to stay asleep.[15]

Drink caffeine only in the morning. Caffeine can also interfere with sleep patterns. We all know that drinking caffeine in the afternoon or evening will often keep us awake at night, so it's best to limit yourself to one cup in the morning if it's something you enjoy.

If you smoke, quit. If you must smoke, avoid doing it within two hours of bedtime, as nicotine is a stimulant.[16]

Go to bed and wake up at the same time every day. There should be an eight-hour window between your set bedtime and wake-up time. For example, if you choose a 10 p.m. bedtime, then your wake-up time is 6 a.m. Stick to this schedule even on weekends, vacations, and holidays if you can.

Optimizing Sleep Quality

When it comes to the quality of sleep, I find that attending to the cross-over between different lifestyle medicine spokes is particularly useful. In addition to being aware of and tapering off your use of substances, here are a few ways to think about sleep management support from elsewhere on the wheel:

- If you must eat something late at night, be sure to keep it light. Eating a heavy meal before bed will keep you up. Try to taper off the amount and richness of your meals through the day—your nighttime self will thank you!

- Engage in thirty minutes of physical activity every day. Using your muscles and increasing blood flow and oxygen during the day contributes to better sleep.

- Stress management practices like those in this book will support more consistent and restful sleep. At the height of my insomnia, I often spent hours each night wide awake in a state of high anxiety. I didn't yet have a regular meditation practice, so I couldn't call on the tools I have now to calm me down, regulate my emotions, and notice and accept my physical reality. Building your practice during the day will serve you well at night.

Technology and Sleep

Finally, I want to address one of the biggest factors affecting the length and quality of sleep today, and that's our 24/7 access to technology. With the mass availability of smartphones, social media, and our endless access to the computer, there is no longer a sharp delineation between work time and personal or leisure time. We check our work email at home, during family dinner, at our child's soccer game. We even stay connected to the stressors and stimulation of work when we're on vacation! Not only do these devices contribute to extra light exposure, but the nonstop connectivity makes them highly addictive as well.

This is no real secret. The tech industry uses the metric of "eyeball hours" in its marketing and advertising plans and actively tries to make content and apps that are "sticky" so that people will be glued to their screens. Climbing screen times are damaging our ability to sleep effectively. In a 2013 study, investigators found the longer participants engaged in screen time, the worse their quality and quantity of sleep.[17]

I know asking anyone to go turn in their phone and live a smartphone-free life is incongruent with life as we know it today. (Even my octogenarian mom is sending me text messages and heart emojis.) But we can become mindful of our practice and work to reduce dependency on this tool.

Here are some suggestions to reduce your smartphone usage:

- Check your screen time in your Settings, so you will be able to see how many minutes or hours you've used the phone for a day or week.

- Turn off notifications from news alerts and all social media outlets.

- Schedule set times to look at your phone, like morning, lunchtime, and late afternoon. Limit these encounters to no more than five minutes each.

- Keep your phone on gray screen. Color stimulates us, so this might especially help those who are really having trouble putting the phone down.

Beyond the minutes and hours lost to our phones, and the extra light that's impeding our sleep, I think there's an opportunity here to look even deeper into our values and how they play out in our everyday behaviors. When it comes to sleep, sometimes we'd like to get away with the least possible amount so we can indulge in more waking hours of achieving, producing, and consuming more. But who benefits from this lifestyle? And at what cost? Prioritizing sleep and respecting the needs of your mind and body will most certainly further the values that align with your larger desires for overall well-being and joyfulness.

Keep It Simple Review

- Your health depends on getting optimal sleep every day.

- Evaluate your current habits to target specific problems with falling asleep, staying asleep, and optimizing the quality of your sleep long term.

- Appreciate how other aspects of lifestyle (other spokes) affect your sleep.

Sleep Diary

As part of my assessment (in addition to taking a thorough medical history and physical examination) I ask patients to complete a sleep diary and to make it as detailed as possible. A sleep diary allows you to collect a bunch of data over the course of a week or two and uncover patterns and possible causes for sleep disturbance. It will also increase your overall awareness of behaviors that play a role in the duration and quality of your sleep. See appendix B for a sleep diary template I use with my patients. (Alternatively, you can create your own version in your journal.)

Action Steps

Here's a quick list of what to look for when designing your sleep plan and reviewing your basic sleep hygiene.

Environment

- Check light levels in your bedroom. If necessary, add light-blocking shades to your windows.

- Check the temperature of the room; it should be comfortably cool.

- Consider the age and comfort level of your mattress and bedding and upgrade them if needed.

- Address any sources contributing to noise which may disrupt your sleep.

Habits

- Try not to eat or drink anything at least two hours before bed.

- Eliminate caffeine, smoking, and other stimulants at least four hours or more before bed.

- Avoid alcohol

- Get at least thirty minutes of exercise per day.

- Turn off all screens at least one hour before bed.

- If you have a habit of watching the evening news, consider whether this is keeping you awake with anxiety; try reading/watching the news in the morning instead.

- Set a regular bedtime and stick with it. Set a corresponding wake-up time in the morning.

Relaxing Rituals

Try any of the following to help wind down in the evening before bed:

- Massage a lavender-infused hand lotion into hands, arms, and elbows.

- Take a warm shower or a bath.

- Practice prayer/gratitude journaling.

- Listen to soft music.

- Practice deep breathing.

- Do a guided sleep meditation.

Substance Intake Awareness

Do the best you can until you know better.
Then when you know better, do better.
—Maya Angelou

I don't have to tell you that smoking, excessive drinking, and abusing drugs are bad for your health. Certainly, you've heard that message before. Besides, if telling people those things were enough to get them to limit their use or stop altogether, it would've already happened.

So while we already know certain substances are harmful to us, what you may not know (and we'll discuss in this chapter) is that other substances, even some that we think of as healthy, including supplements, vitamins, and herbs touted as cures or wellness boosters, can be dangerous too. Still, it's one thing to ingest substances that we think are good for us, and quite another to keep on using things that we know will impact our health in negative ways. Yet smoking and vaping, as well as alcohol and drug abuse, clearly persist. Why?

There are many reasons for this, of course, and a full discussion is beyond the scope of this book. It's certainly safe to say that some of us are likelier to engage in these harmful behaviors than others, and a number of variables can contribute to this tendency, including our genes, our personal history and family experiences, our psychological mindset, and our cultural norms. Much has been written about who's most affected by addictive substances, and we're discovering more about this all the time.

At its heart, whether it be tobacco, alcohol, painkillers, or illegal recreational drugs, there is a powerful internal driver in some people who seek these escapes. There are competing theories as to why we turn to substances. Do we seek pleasure or a momentary release from pain? Or both? What is at the root of addiction and substance abuse?

The self-medication hypothesis, introduced in 1985, maintains that psychological suffering is the driving force behind the development of dependence.[1] Substances offer relief from painful experiences—they transport us away from our negative perceptions, offering temporary ease from life's difficult challenges. In my work with patients, I've found this is often, but not always, one of the main reasons people turn to substances.

While the reasons we might start are complex and varied, the reasons we continue are fairly straightforward. Addictive substances hijack and rewire the limbic system of the brain, our reward center. They flood it with an intense reward (pleasure, release from pain) that often wears off quickly, leaving a crater of need in its place. Through this feedback loop of need and reward, the brain builds up tolerance to a substance, so that it requires a higher dosage to get the same level of reward or even to feel normal. In addition to the powerful changes in the brain and body, dependence builds through behavioral changes. Maintaining access to the substance takes up time and energy, and behaviors that used to be rewarding, such as a walk in the park or connecting with a loved one, cannot compete with the ability of the substance to flood the brain and body with the desired reward.

This powerful physical and psychological cycle is very difficult to break. Physicians know this, and yet even health-care professionals have been drawn into one of the most destructive addiction epidemics in modern history: the opioid epidemic. We'll get to that. But first, let's take a look at the roles tobacco and alcohol have played in our society and what this may mean in your own life.

Tobacco

Cultural acceptance is an incredibly powerful variable in human behavior. Consider how, in the past fifty years, smoking has gone from being considered cool and fashionable to being thought of as distasteful and dangerous. We can thank scientists for establishing the risks of smoking and secondhand smoke, leaders in government for limiting where you can smoke and increasing taxes on tobacco, and massive educational campaigns for accelerating the shift away from societal acceptance of tobacco use. This took plenty of hard work and is in some ways a model for what we can accomplish via public awareness of lifestyle medicine. The numbers show that we have made great strides in this area, from near half the U.S. population of adults smoking in the 1960s, to most recent estimates at 13.7 percent.[2] This is very favorable news, but in my opinion it is still 13.7 percent too many.

Approximately thirty-four million Americans smoke, and regrettably this includes many of our most vulnerable residents, including the uninsured, psychologically impaired, disabled, and those living below the poverty line. On a global scale, the WHO informs us that tobacco kills more than eight million people a year, with the great majority living in low- and middle-income countries. Smoking alone accounts for 15 percent of all deaths worldwide.[3] Heart disease, lung cancer, and chronic obstructive pulmonary disease (COPD) top the list of causes of death for smokers.

Tobacco is most commonly being sold and marketed to those who have the least access to health care and the lowest level of education.[4] The best weapon we have to curtail smoking on a universal scale is education, as it helps reduce new users. But as mentioned earlier, education isn't enough. The harder aspect is helping those already addicted to break the habit. This applies to every substance addiction: stopping is far harder than never beginning in the first place, and sustaining that abstinence is hardest of all. Clinical studies report the greatest smoking cessation success rates are achieved when patients receive a combination of counseling and medication. There are prescription medications approved by the FDA for this indication, as well as nicotine replacement therapies like the patch, nasal spray, gum, or lozenges, all of which have been shown to have some efficacy. Options such as these, which further enhance the likelihood of success when quitting, should be discussed with a physician or clinician who is an expert in smoking cessation, as they are the best qualified to assess whether or not someone is a suitable candidate. To be clear, I am in no way against prescription medication in general—quite the contrary. For me, optimal health is an ongoing personal process guided by trusted medical professionals, and any substances should be taken under careful supervision, along with robust lifestyle interventions when appropriate. I'm including a list of free and accessible resources available to those seeking support at the end of this chapter.

Alcohol

When it comes to cigarettes, the message is clear: there's no safe level of tobacco use. Likewise, of course, with illicit drugs. Yet when we turn our attention to alcohol, society's acceptance is quite different from tobacco use. Alcohol often plays a role in socializing and celebrating and is even thought of as a social lubricant, something that relaxes us or "takes the edge off."

The average person does not consider alcohol damaging to their health. In fact, many people believe that alcohol has health benefits. This is partly thanks to conclusions like that of the American Heart Association, which states that moderate intake is acceptable, and actually even states moderate intake has been associated with cardiovascular benefits.[5] Nonetheless, the AHA falls short of recommending drinking alcohol for heart health, instead advising patients to consume a healthy diet to maximally protect their hearts. We now know that any benefits gained from red wine can also be achieved simply by eating red grapes, and any cardiovascular benefits could more easily be added by walking an extra few minutes a day. Regrettably in past cancer prevention guidelines, the American Cancer Society also accepted moderate intake for those who do choose to drink, but in their most recent updated recommendations published in June 2020, they added "It is best not to drink alcohol." This was a significant and important step by the organization and frankly reflects what the science is telling us.[6]

Part of the problem with alcohol is that when it comes to defining appropriate usage, even the federal guidelines are ambiguous at best and harmful at worst. For instance, the CDC guidelines state that "if alcohol is consumed, it should be consumed in 'moderation.' " The guidelines then go on to define moderation as "up to one alcoholic drink per day for women, and two alcoholic drinks per day for men."[7] One obvious ambiguity is that the size of "one alcoholic drink" varies depending on the kind of alcohol you're consuming. So according to these guidelines, that's 12 ounces of beer, 8 ounces of malt liquor, 5 ounces of wine, or 1.5 ounces of distilled spirits. Consider how these guidelines measure up in real life. For instance, many large wine glasses can easily hold 10 ounces, which means one glass of wine at dinner is not in fact moderation for women, but double that amount.

These guidelines beg an additional question: Is daily or even regular drinking healthy?

It is not. My challenge for you is to rethink your need to drink. See if you can skip the next several instances when you would normally include alcohol as a part of your routine. As you evaluate your drinking habits, consider whether you are using alcohol as stress relief, as a sleep aid, or to enhance your ability to make social connections. This is an important exercise to gain insight on your current habits. Remember, our goal in lifestyle medicine is optimal health, and this includes making sure you aren't using a substance like alcohol to do for you what you truly are capable of doing on your own.

While many people who drink alcohol regularly don't meet the medical definition of alcohol use disorder (AUD) or what was once referred to as alcohol dependence, I do feel it's important to point out that one of the most common characteristics of AUD may be denial. In other words, unlike the diseases of cancer, diabetes, or MS, someone suffering from AUD will often deny they have a problem, even when confronted with a mountain of evidence suggesting that alcohol is impeding their overall well-being. Sadly, denial of a problem is often the response when I tell a patient that their drinking habits are well beyond what any reasonable person would consider as normal. Perhaps you remember the patient Jim from chapter 4. He admitted to me that he drank heavily "most nights," that he often became verbally abusive when he did so, and that his ex-wife cited his drinking as one of the main reasons she left the marriage. Yet despite this, when I asked him if he thought alcohol was a problem, he replied without hesitation, "Absolutely not! I can quit anytime."

That's why I say that when it comes to alcohol use, awareness is key. Addiction is both a cunning and powerful foe, and no one starts out drinking or using drugs with the intent to develop a problem. Instead, it sneaks up on them, and knowing when you're in trouble is the first step in being able to seek and accept help. This requires recognition and honesty about your own usage and very often input from a family member or friend witnessing the behavior. Luckily, there are a wide range of treatments and services to help people stop drinking, from inpatient treatment facilities to outpatient programs and recovery support groups. If you or someone you love has a problem with alcohol, please seek help. If you are a family member or loved one of someone suffering from AUD also consider reaching out for support for yourself. This is one spoke on the lifestyle medicine wheel that it is almost impossible to address alone.

Prescription Painkillers and the Opioid Epidemic

Let's talk about prescription painkillers. Beginning in the late 1990s, pharmaceutical companies began a massive marketing effort to convince physicians that a patient's pain must be treated. In their view, of course, medical professionals should treat pain with prescribed painkillers. Every patient who came into the clinic was asked to evaluate their pain on a scale of 1 to 10, with 1 being mild pain and 10 being the worst pain possible.

Even organizations like the Joint Commission, which accredits hospitals, created standards in 2001 in response to what was perceived to be a national outcry about "the widespread problem of underassessment and undertreatment of pain."[8] This seems to have originated not with patients themselves, but in the marketing departments of pharmaceutical companies eager to capitalize on a universal human aversion to pain and a cultural desire to be comfortable.

Physicians were compelled to treat pain, and companies assured them that their patients would not become addicted to pain relievers. This gave physicians a green light to prescribe more freely and led to widespread misuse and abuse of opioids, which are in fact highly addictive. By 2017, the Department of Health and Human Services declared a public health emergency. Two million Americans are currently living with an opioid use disorder, and 130 people a day are dying in this epidemic.[9] We will be battling this complex crisis for decades to come.

Pain Can Be a Message

While I'm clearly disappointed by what appears to have been a manufactured movement to quell universal pain for financial expediency, I don't mean to imply that pain isn't real or that we should ignore it. You probably know this from experience, and I certainly do, that ignoring pain can really backfire. So many of us were told as kids—particularly young athletes—to "power through" pain, which, as we have seen in several instances throughout this book, can be another example of an unhelpful cultural norm.

Pain almost always has a message for us.

There are certainly instances of emotional growth that can and often be interpreted as painful—ending a significant relationship that we know we must is a good example of this. Furthermore, major life changes in general often require us to go outside of what feels comfortable in order to learn new skills or mature. But in all of these instances, we can be consoled that some kinds of discomfort are an indicator that we are growing in positive ways.

On the other hand, pain can also be a warning or a profound indicator of something we need to investigate. Pain can serve as a signal that we are out of alignment with some aspect of ourselves, either physically or emotionally. Physical pain can be an indicator of injury or the onset of illness and the need to seek immediate medical attention. Emotional pain may be part of a larger process, such as sadness or grief. In these cases, when we ignore or try to "power through" this kind of pain, the suffering almost always gets worse, sometimes becoming debilitating.

It's these instances that are often the impetus of a drug, alcohol, or smoking addiction cycle. Since many of these substances are depressants, they can help mute certain kinds of physical and emotional pain for a time, but they can't heal the root cause of pain. So when the effects of these substances wear off, the pain returns and feels even worse, initiating a cycle of increasing dependency.

I want to be clear that physical pain is something you always want to be sure to check out with your doctor as soon as possible. However, on an emotional level, how do we know the difference between discomfort that signals growth and learning and the kind of pain that warns us that something is out of balance and must be addressed? The most direct way I know of to make this distinction is through mindful awareness. Here is yet another example of how the lifestyle medicine spokes interact with and support one another. In this case, mindfulness involves checking in with our emotions in the present moment and also being able to observe the perceptions and self-talk occurring in our minds. If we turn to substances to change our perception of ourselves or to overcome negative self-talk, that's an indication we are offtrack. This self-talk might sound like statements such as "This situation is never going to get better" or "I'm not strong enough, good enough, etc."

I certainly do not have all the answers, but I know that there is pain (both emotional and physical) that can be managed or even prevented by optimizing all of our lifestyle medicine spokes. And, as I have tried to make clear throughout this book, lifestyle medicine is not a replacement but rather a long-awaited addition to the profound gains in health and wellness experienced worldwide thanks to advances in medicine. The combination of lifestyle practices and traditional medicine holds the greatest promise.

Vitamins and Supplements

It might seem strange to include vitamins and supplements in the same chapter with a discussion about the dangers of drugs, alcohol, and smoking. But from a lifestyle medicine perspective, I feel that this is where they belong. That's because often the impulse behind the use of vitamins and supplements can come from the desire to take a kind of shortcut or find an easy way out.

That was what I did when I turned to taking supplements in 2007, and I ended up in the hospital as a result.

I was three years into my lifestyle change and feeling strong, fit, and confident. I was lifting weights three to four times a week and beginning to run distances. I was free of medication, eating plenty of plants, and sleeping well, and, best of all, my MS was quiet. I loved my work, colleagues, and patients.

The only drawback was my commute to work. One day, my nanny called about an emergency with my son, who was six at the time. He ended up being fine, but it had taken me a full hour to get home to him, and this left me shaken. Because of this, I decided to accept a job offer closer to my home.

My new position was stressful, and I felt like a fish out of water. I justified the move by reminding myself that I was now closer to my children, could work from home some days, and was bringing in a considerably higher income. I tried incorporating aspects of my old job into the new one, offering health and wellness classes and walking groups to my corporate colleagues. I pushed down the pain I felt, chalking it up to growing pains and the challenges of a new environment. But I became more and more unhappy, and six months into the job I noticed that my energy level and mood were starting to sag and my stress level was way up.

Rather than address the stress directly, I began to search for something to keep my energy elevated. I read a book written by a board-certified, Ivy League–trained physician who enumerated the many benefits of consuming his recommended line of supplements. I convinced myself that this might pull me out of my slump, and I thought it couldn't hurt to try.

After several months of his expensive routine, which entailed swallowing lots of large pills throughout the day, I grew weaker and more unwell. I began to experience nausea, even vomiting on several occasions. Initially, I didn't make the connection between these pills and how bad I was feeling. Instead I was worried that my MS symptoms might be returning.

Finally, I felt bad enough to call a friend, who also happened to be my gynecologist, and mentioned the relentless fatigue and nausea I was experiencing. She was convinced I was pregnant and asked me to come into the office that day. The pregnancy test was negative, so she ordered several blood tests. The following day she called, very alarmed. My liver enzymes were sky-high, and I needed to go to the emergency room—immediately.

Once I saw those results, I looked in the mirror and realized that I was jaundiced. The white portion of my eyes was notably yellow, a clear sign of liver disease. I was in acute liver failure.

How could I have missed this?

I was admitted to the hospital, and after many tests and questions turned up nothing, a liver biopsy was ordered. The results read *panacinar hepatitis Zone 3 necrosis*. Necrosis means dead tissue; my liver was dying! The liver biopsy slides were complicated to interpret, so they were sent to an expert at the Mayo Clinic, who wrote back that the liver damage was "strongly suggestive of a drug reaction."

But I wasn't taking any drugs—I was only taking supplements. Most of us don't consider supplements "drugs," yet they are—and they can be far more dangerous than most of us understand. It turned out that the supplements I was taking were responsible for my liver problems.

It took more than six months to recover from this illness, and it could have been much worse, with the very real possibility of irreparable liver failure, liver transplantation, or even death. Examples like mine are not uncommon and often don't end as well.

While many of us are aware of the potential side effects associated with prescription drugs, there is a dangerous perception in our culture that supplements are generally harmless because they are "natural" or because they are widely available at any number of health food stores and websites. But supplements can affect our body in powerful ways, and like prescription drugs, they can also have serious side effects. Supplements, which include vitamins, herbal extracts, amino acids, probiotics, protein powders, and many other compounds in an array of forms and combinations, make up a massive, highly profitable, and generally unregulated industry, and we need to be aware of this when we make choices about what we ingest.

In addition to adopting a healthy, informed approach to prescription drugs, it's vital that we do so with all supplements as well. Always check with your doctor before you begin any new supplement or prescription drug.

I am not opposed to necessary medications and medical interventions, and certainly vitamins are sometimes needed to correct an imbalance or treat a deficiency. For example, vitamin B_{12} and vitamin D are mentioned earlier in this book, and they are both supplements I will recommend if warranted.

The Power of Love and Lifestyle Medicine

In summary, I'd like to add that if you struggle with tobacco, alcohol, or any other addictive substances, you may have already tried to quit countless times with no success. First, I want to validate your experience and your efforts. Addictive substances can maintain a powerful hold on us physically, psychologically, and socially. Anyone working to change these habits knows how difficult it can be to do so. The average person has to try quitting several times before they finally achieve success, and maintaining abstinence is a lifelong commitment. The good news is that your next attempt is *not diminished* by how many times you've tried in the past. Today may be your last quit date. There are many tools available that can help you on your road to successfully overcoming addiction.

One tool that lifestyle medicine offers is self-love. What I mean is that although I could easily have filled this chapter with terrifying lists of the dangers of substance abuse, my own experience tells me that the most meaningful, sustainable habit changes always come from embracing a positive perspective. Even my decision to reject MS medication ultimately came from a positive desire to claim a quality of life that felt sustainable to me—as free from pain and suffering and in line with my values as possible.

Lifestyle medicine's primary catalyst for change is love. Prominent lifestyle medicine leader Dr. Dean Ornish reminds us that we achieve lasting change not by "*fear of death,* but instead by the *joy of living.*" It makes sense, if you think about it. When we experience fear—or fear's offshoots such as anger, shame, or worthlessness—we are sapped of our energy and our well-being is worn down. Love, on the other hand, with its attendant feelings of gratitude, generosity, forgiveness, and empathy, will always *replenish* our emotional and physical health. Feeling good in this way makes change desirable and sustainable, even when we encounter inevitable obstacles. That is my hope and wish for you.

Keep It Simple Review

- Choose love over fear.

- Tune in to emotional pain and practice interpreting its source through mindfulness.

- Notice your own substance issues and work to address their influence on your health and well-being.

Envision the Joy of Living Substance-Free

Some of us are simply not aware of our reliance on substances day to day. Much like a food or sleep diary, it can be helpful to simply record, for a week or a month, how much you are using things like tobacco, alcohol, supplements, prescriptions, or other substances. This gives you and your doctor some baseline information from which you can evaluate where you are now and begin a treatment plan if necessary.

Smoking—Did You Know?

When it comes to smoking, here's something I find inspiring: You don't have to wait long before you reap tangible health benefits from tobacco cessation. In just a short amount of time, things start getting better. Check out these facts from the CDC:

- 20 minutes after you quit, your heart rate decreases.

- 12 hours after you quit, the level of carbon monoxide in your blood returns to normal.

- 2 weeks to 3 months after you quit, your risk of dying from a heart attack begins to drop, and your lung function begins to improve.

- 1 to 9 months after you quit, your cough and shortness of breath decrease.

- 1 year after you quit, your risk of heart disease is half that of an active smoker.

- 5 years after you quit, your risk of stroke is that of a nonsmoker.

- 10 years after you quit, your lung cancer risk is half of a smoker's.

- 15 years after you quit, your risk of a heart attack is back to that of a nonsmoker.[10]

Resources for Quitting

Telephone quit line counseling (e.g., 1-800-QUIT-NOW) is a great place to start for those who are contemplating a future quit date or who are ready today.

The American Heart Association, American Cancer Society, and the Centers for Disease Control and Prevention also offer invaluable resources and even provide planning tools and access to coaches to create a road map that best serves individuals.

Smokefree.gov offers daily text messaging to support patients, even tailoring texts to resonate with different segments of the population, such as women, teenagers, veterans, Spanish-speaking individuals, and so on. This is a tool I have found to be very effective with my patients to help keep them on track and support their quit attempt.

For alcohol and drug cessation, the CDC website offers videos, infographics, podcasts, and webinars, free and accessible to all, and you can learn more about 12-step programs, including where to find a meeting near you, by visiting Alcoholics Anonymous at www.aa.org or Narcotics Anonymous at www.na.org. Meeting attendance at both of these organizations is free.

The Healing Power of Human Connection

Alone, we can do so little; together, we can do so much.
—Helen Keller

On October 17, 1995, twin girls were born twelve weeks prematurely. With steep odds against their survival, and each weighing about two pounds, the girls were placed in separate incubators in the neonatal intensive care unit. This was the routine standard of care at the time, as physicians wanted to protect both babies against the risk of infection. In this case, one of the twins seemed to thrive, while her smaller sister struggled with difficulty breathing, unstable body temperature, and heart problems. The weaker baby continued to deteriorate and was placed in critical condition in early November. Witnessing their daughter's decline, the twins' parents desperately sought any remedy. A nurse named Gayle Kasparian suggested something she had heard was practiced in Europe. She proposed placing the girls together in one incubator. What followed was miraculous. Immediately, the stronger twin wrapped her arm around her fragile smaller sister. In a short time, the frail twin's blood oxygen, heart rate, and body temperature improved. Today, the twins are healthy adults who remain lovingly bonded.[1]

Their story changed the course of neonatal medicine, as it is now considered reasonable, and even beneficial, to co-bed sets of twins. We don't fully understand how the benefits work. Is it coincidence that the child suddenly flourished when cuddled by her sibling, or is there a way to prove that her recovery was linked to their being together? How can we measure the health benefit of healing touch and human connections in general?

From a medical perspective, it's hard to design a study for this, yet there is a growing body of evidence supporting the importance of social connections. Social interactions have been shown to strongly influence psychological and physical health outcomes, as well as survival and the ability to thrive.[2]

I want to take a moment here to underline once again the complexity of overall health. Everything fits together, and when it comes to the spokes on our lifestyle medicine wheel, balance is important. Social connection is an essential piece of the larger health puzzle that my colleagues in medicine very often ignore or minimize. It's poetic to say that someone "died of a broken heart," but the truth is that loneliness and isolation are real health dangers. Fortunately, meaningful connection and a sense of belonging are also strong medicine. Like nutrition, exercise, stress, and sleep, the impact of social connection on our health and well-being is influenced by many factors, including the sum of our experiences and our baseline physical and psychological makeup. Simply put, we cannot ignore the compelling objective evidence of the merits of connectedness.

We Are Social Creatures

This sense of belonging is one of our most basic human needs—from the moment we're born all the way through to the final moments of our lives. We are social creatures; human brains and bodies have evolved to maximize love and belonging. Not only does it feel good to feel connected, it fuels a wide range of behaviors that build over time to support a better, healthier, and longer life on an individual level—and stronger and better functioning communities on a societal level.

Various studies have found many benefits of social connection in health outcomes:

- Protecting against inflammation, which is connected to the vast majority of chronic diseases.[3]

- Lowering the likelihood of individuals to be obese, have high blood pressure, or suffer from metabolic dysregulation.[4]

- Promoting a healthier lifestyle, including consuming more vegetables and engaging in more physical activity.[5]

- Delaying memory loss among elderly Americans.[6]

- Raising survival rates for women with breast cancer.[7]

- Lowering rates of fatal heart attacks.[8]

On the other hand, how do those who describe themselves as suffering from loneliness fare? It turns out that feeling isolated is catastrophic to our well-being.[9] UC Berkeley's Greater Good website summarizes the dangers in this way:

> On the flipside, social isolation and loneliness are bad for our health. The more socially isolated older adults are, the more they tend to be inactive, smoke, and have higher blood pressure and other risk factors for heart disease. Several studies suggest that socially isolated adults also have an increased risk of death.[10]

The takeaways are crystal clear: the more meaningful folks we have in our social circles, and the more regular connection we enjoy, the greater our personal health benefits. As a variety of factors in our modern world erode certain aspects of social connection, it's essential to take a careful look at the importance of this spoke, for ourselves and society as a whole. Elderly people, for example, are likelier to be alone and isolated. As our older population grows, the effect on public health is only anticipated to rise.[11]

As with every major area of health and well-being in this book, my focus here is to give you a simple, practical approach to transforming your health and your life. With a little attentiveness and a willingness to try, you can vastly increase the reach and quality of your social connections and bolster your health and well-being in so many ways.

Circles of Influence

Consider for a moment what a map of your connections to the people and communities in your life might look like. Maybe it's something like the illustration below.

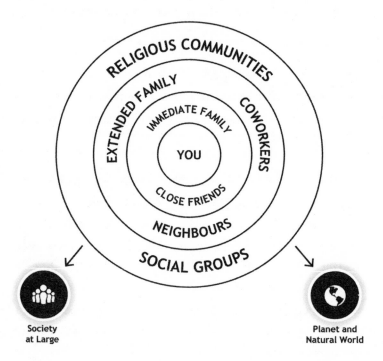

This is only one way to look at social connection, and in reality these boundaries are much more flexible, like a web. A web is a good metaphor indeed, as you can almost feel a pull or a tug when something is happening in any of your circles. A profound loss, an illness, or a joyful event can send vibrations to you and everyone else in your web. A friend's school community recently suffered the loss of a child to gun violence, and it ripped a hole in their shared web. Thanks to the connection and the commitment of the community, however, families and friends rallied around the boy's family, bringing comfort and material support when it was most needed. That loss will always be felt and remembered, but the web as a whole was in some ways strengthened by the tragic experience.

Take a look at the inner circles of this map. When it comes to your immediate family in the first circle, and your extended family and close friends in the second, how strong do these connections feel to you right now? Be honest. Just as in previous assessments we've done, a forthright sense of where you are now is essential to figuring out where you want to be. Many of us might find that these social connections are not as strong as we might like, or that we unintentionally take them for granted or feel so overwhelmed by our professional lives that we don't invest the time and energy we would like to in our family relationships and friendships. We may also be in the midst of a painful separation or ongoing feud. These take a toll on our health as well.

Here, we can look to the blue zones for guidance. In chapter 2, we touched briefly on the health and lifestyle examples of these particular places across the globe, which have the highest incidence of people living into their hundreds and markedly healthy and happy populations. Strong social ties are a vital part of the wellness of these communities.

Let's return to the Okinawan custom of *moais,* groups of friends unrelated by blood who remain devoted to caring for each other over a lifetime. In light of the findings from studies on social connection, it makes sense that such a practice would benefit longevity.[12] The blue zones share a tendency to prioritize close human bonds, particularly cherishing family ties. Parents and grandparents often live in the same home with children and grandchildren, and families are built around long-lasting marriages. Families in these areas also tend to stay close to home, often living in the same town their whole lives. In the United States and European countries, on the other hand, it's quite common for extended families to spread far across continents or even across the planet.

In much of the world, getting older means being at greater risk of social isolation, but when that happens, it's a missed opportunity, as these elders have much to teach the younger generations and along with close friendships can fortify the second ring of our circle. When the older members of our family share the same kinds of values that we do, they can become role models to our kids, confidants to us, and encourage our health and well-being.

It's important to tend to the outer circles as well—our neighbors, coworkers, faith communities, medical support groups, addiction recovery groups, local governments, and more. Everyone has their own individual map of influence, and the web changes organically over time. If you're dealing with a coworker who is in turn caring for a sick parent, you can strengthen your overall social web by checking in and offering a listening ear. This builds trust, the gold standard of social currency. Furthermore, small, regular social interactions are far better at building and affirming trust than big, life-changing or dramatic moments. Think of the people in your circle who know your children's names or who call to see how you're feeling if you miss an event or don't show up to work. These seemingly little things build up your overall well-being in powerful ways.

Now that we've mapped our social connections, let's take a look at how we might strengthen that web, so we can get the most out of this essential spoke on our lifestyle medicine wheel.

Finding Work-Life Balance

Like it or not, our culture values wealth and prosperity, which we're encouraged to pursue even at the cost of individual health and well-being. This is one of the ways our web can get out of alignment. Even Merriam-Webster's definition of the American dream speaks to materialism and acquisition, calling it "an American social ideal that stresses egalitarianism and especially material prosperity."[13]

In the United States, acquiring wealth is often the chief metric for success. As we have seen in other spokes of the lifestyle medicine wheel, advertisers formulate and manipulate these wealth and success standards to sell their products. We are made to feel lacking so that we're primed to acquire more. Of course, there's nothing wrong with entrepreneurship and building wealth, and we live in a country with incredible freedom of choice and opportunity—but if we spend too much time on the acquisition of "stuff," that often comes at the expense of our social connections. Remember the sixty-one-year-old patient Jim I mentioned in chapter 4? As I got to know him better, he confided in me that his biggest regret was spending so much time building his business that he neglected his wife, children, and other close connections in the process. Unfortunately, I hear this type of thing a lot. Not only can we not get that time back with our loved ones, but this behavior can contribute to our health problems as well.

In my own life, I'd always aspired to buy a nice home in a lovely neighborhood, to earn enough for my kids to go to top universities, and to retire in comfort. I knew that as a physician this would mean working long hours and returning to full-time work within a few months of my kids being born. I didn't question this plan until everything changed on the morning of 9/11.

I was working in New York state at the time and had dropped my nine-month-old son at day care before traveling twenty miles down to my clinic at the Castle Point VA. As I began to see patients, the news spread across the facility. Before I knew it, all the television screens had turned to the tragedy. My first thought was that I needed to get to my son. But the administration told us we would not be allowed to leave and that we should prepare to treat any incoming injured. My husband, also a physician, was on call for labor and delivery in New Jersey and could not leave either.

Like every doctor that day, I held on to my responsibility to care for those suffering—we did not yet know that there were more fatalities than survivors. That night, I wept with relief, grateful to have gotten home with my son Nicholas, and I had no desire to go back to work the next day—or possibly ever. Of course, I did go to work the next day, but I asked to go to part-time and eventually made the switch so that I could spend more time with my son. The experience of 9/11 left me and everyone I knew considering our own mortality and reevaluating our priorities.

Over time, however, that feeling faded and life got busy. Within a couple of years I had returned to a full-time, hectic schedule, eager to make more money. In 2012, I decided that I needed to focus on my family, and I stepped down from a stressful job and started my own private practice focusing exclusively on lifestyle medicine.

At first, the loss of income felt worrisome and personally demeaning. I had based so much of my self-worth on my ability to make money. In time, though, I came to realize that I had made the right decision for myself and my family. I was able to create a work environment where I could see patients for five or six hours a day and still be able to be there for pickup, after-school activities, and preparing family meals. I was managing my MS with lifestyle medicine at this time as well, so having extra hours in the day to exercise and support a self-care routine felt essential. Reducing my work hours was one of the best decisions I ever made. In retrospect, I wish I'd done it earlier.

This is not to say that mothers and fathers who work outside the home should feel regret or guilt. In general, I find shame and judgment to be unhelpful, and I try to remember that I know very little about anyone else's personal situation. In my case, it turned out that fortifying my web of social connection involved choosing to stay home more. I didn't make this decision lightly, though I feel fortunate that this was an option for me. I also understand that many parents simply don't have the economic ability to make this choice.

In our society, finding work-life balance can be a challenge. But we can assess our daily routines and see if the time and energy we are spending is in alignment with our values and goals. For me, seeing that eight to ten hours of every weekday were going to my coworkers and patients and only two to three were going to my son at a time when I knew he was making huge developmental steps wasn't going to work.

I invite you to check in with yourself and feel out your current investment in your close family and friend relationships. Do they feel strong and supportive? Do you invest "quantity time" and not just "quality time"? Spending quality time with loved ones is wonderful, for sure, but it's just as important if not more so to engage in regular—maybe boring—care and connection with your partner or spouse, your kids or grandkids, the elders in your life, and your closest friends. Daily or weekly connections go a long way in fostering deep, trusting relationships.

This is not to say you won't continue to evaluate, make adjustments, and recalibrate your goals and behaviors over time; balance is achieved in motion, with many tiny, constant adjustments. Remember that it's almost impossible to balance on a bicycle while standing still, but begin to move forward with a little push and balance becomes possible—even easy.

Asking for Help

Hardships can be an obstacle to increasing social connection. When we're going through hard times, we often withdraw from family, friends, and neighbors. This might not be a conscious choice, but anyone who has experienced a financial, personal, or health crisis probably knows what I mean. We might feel ashamed or like we don't have anyone we can trust or lean on for help. We might be influenced by a damaging expectation that we have to put up a good front or remain self-sufficient at all costs. I certainly felt this way as a young doctor, and it's one of the reasons I strove to hide my illness from my patients and colleagues for so long. I was supposed to be the helper, not the one needing help. I realized, however, that this view was inconsistent with who I wanted to be, because it was fundamentally judgmental about those I wanted to help. In other words, if I thought it was so terrible to be vulnerable, what did that say about my own patients? Were they terrible for being open and honest about needing assistance? Of course not! I learned to extend the same kindness and care to myself as I was able to access for my patients. This meant that I learned—finally—to ask for and receive help.

Acknowledging Our Interconnectedness

Social connections lead to shared behavior. You could even say that the actions and attitudes of those around us are infectious. A 2009 *New York Times* article described the landmark Framingham Heart Study (FHS), which began in 1948 as a government-funded effort to understand the true cause of heart disease. The article focused on the work of two social scientists, Nicholas Christakis and James Fowler, who studied the immense FHS database and concluded that how we behave in our community directly impacts the health of the people in our immediate circle and even those two or three degrees away:

> By analyzing the Framingham data, Christakis and Fowler say, they have for the first time found some solid basis for a potentially powerful theory in epidemiology: that good behaviors—like quitting smoking or staying slender or being happy—pass from friend to friend almost as if they were contagious viruses. The Framingham participants, the data suggested, influenced one another's health just by socializing. And the same was true of bad behaviors—clusters of friends appeared to "infect" each other with obesity, unhappiness and smoking.[14]

In other words, people influence others' health by simply engaging in social interactions.[15]

Christakis and Fowler found that when a Framingham resident became obese, his or her friends were 57 percent likelier to become obese too. And if a friend of a friend became obese, the Framingham resident was about 20 percent likelier to become obese—even if the connecting friend didn't gain a single pound. This makes sense, if you think about it; people are connected, and therefore our health is connected as well.

Since we know that social connections bolster both negative and positive behaviors, it's important to choose your groups wisely to maximize your own personal transformation goals. If you've noticed that a friend isn't supportive of some of the changes you're making, maybe try to include them in activities you know you both would enjoy, to keep that connection going while fostering positive change as well. Give people the chance to grow with you. If you've determined that you need to create some space, that's OK too. On the flip side, consider how your actions and attitude may be rubbing off on your friends. Are you positive, supportive, and as encouraging of your friends' successes as you are of your own? Do you make as much of an effort to connect as they do?

Practicing Forgiveness

I'd like to wrap up this chapter with a few words on forgiveness. My lifestyle medicine approach requires that I do a thorough evaluation with new patients, including social connections. Far too often, as I counsel patients and families, they talk to me about ongoing familial conflicts, anger, and resentment. What I have found is that as humans we often hold on to our deepest grudges and offenses against family members—after all, those closest to us often have the most power to inflict hurt. These disputes might go on for a long time, at enormous cost to everyone.

One of my patients recently told me that she and her brother had not spoken to each other for years. When I asked her why, she responded, "He's a jerk." But as we talked, her sense of regret began to come through. At one point, she told me, they were very close. I encouraged her to share some of those good memories. I was surprised as she went on, smiling as she shared one loving encounter after another. Then I asked if she could describe the inciting event—the moment when things turned sour. She paused, her eyes filled with tears, and she said, "Lots of little things, really. I don't have one specific thing; I just feel like he was never there for me when I needed him."

I've heard similar stories from other patients and seen how conflicts that remain unforgiven often leave in their wake a void of pain and solitude. Grudges and feuds take the joy out of life, and prevent us from deepening our connections to the people in our innermost circle. I think this is why so many religious and spiritual traditions all over the world encourage the practice of forgiveness. We have learned that strengthening the depth and quality of our connections with others serves to reduce our risk of disease and support our own longevity. Forgiveness is one of the most direct and powerful paths to access these benefits.

I want to be clear—forgiveness doesn't mean being "nice" or allowing yourself to be hurt or staying in an abusive or unhealthy situation. In fact, forgiveness can be an important aspect of self-care, as you realize that you deserve to be loved and treated well. Everyone makes mistakes, but if there is a pattern of bad behavior, it's important to stand up for yourself and create some distance in whatever way makes the most sense. In these cases perhaps most of all, forgiving another person for past hurts—whether or not they "deserve" forgiveness—can be a profoundly healing and transformational experience, as you let go of the pain on your own terms and move on.

Is there someone out there for whom you've held a grudge or resentment for years? What if you were to reach out to this person? Or if that's not best or even possible, can you imagine an encounter with them in your mind? Start with a clear and generous intention, something along the lines of, "I know we've been distant for a long time, and I've felt guilty and sad about it. Would you be opposed to sharing how you feel with me?" Own your part of the story, including any mistakes you've made or hurt you've caused. Commit to listening to their side of things. What would that feel like? It's probably a little scary to think about. What if they reject your kindness? What if it makes you feel inferior, embarrassed, or foolish? Let me assure you that regardless of how the other person reacts, this act of forgiveness and connection will be a big win for you. Even if you are not able to repair your relationship, forgiveness will empower you to let go and move on, rather than being a victim stuck in your past pain.

Remember, no matter what happens, you can always call on your mindfulness practice to see and experience things as they are, not as you wish them to be. When a conflict arises with family or close friends, the only thing you can control is your response. Feel your feelings, acknowledge them, and cherish your loved ones as they are. Your love, kindness, and acceptance trump all.

In my view, we build the closest bonds of social connection through our vulnerability. Fred Rogers of *Mr. Rogers' Neighborhood* is a hero of mine, and I recall that a high school student once wrote to him asking, "What was the greatest event in American history?" He replied: "I can't say. However, I suspect that like so many 'great' events, it was something very simple and very quiet with little or no fanfare (such as someone forgiving someone else for a deep hurt that eventually changed the course of history)."[16]

Forgiveness is a critical and sometimes misunderstood part of living a whole and connected life. We can all think of times when we've been hurt by others or have hurt others ourselves, and our culture tells us that forgiveness is important. But usually our awareness of the power of forgiveness stops there. Forgiveness is not about pretending that what happened is OK or "letting someone off the hook" for hurting you. Instead, it's about letting go of the way that past hurt is continuing to hurt you. Forgiving others means that you are releasing *yourself* in order to move forward.

Of course, this can be a challenging process for many of us. Luckily, there are exercises available to us to strengthen our "forgiveness muscles," and I've included some of these at the end of this chapter. I hope you will consider them a part of your journey as you foster strong social bonds with your family, your friends, and your community.

Keep It Simple Review

- Map your connections—who makes up your circle of influence?

- Fortify the web—address any obstacles to deeper, more meaningful connections.

- Try something new—use the exercise below to find new ways to connect.

- Don't underestimate the power of forgiveness.

Engaging with Your Community

While seniors are at particular risk for social isolation, people of all ages and from all walks of life benefit from staying engaged socially.[17] Here are twenty activities to increase your social connections with folks who are similarly engaged in positive behaviors:

1. Take a class in something you are passionate about.

2. Learn how to play an instrument or learn a new language in a group class.

3. Join a local book club.

4. Join a walking group.

5. Sing in the church choir.

6. Audition for a role in a community theater production.

7. Volunteer at a local animal shelter.

8. Mentor a young person.

9. Start a community-wide awareness program, like recycling, planting a garden, or cleaning up a local park.

10. Volunteer at the local senior citizens home.

11. Invite three or four friends to be part of your official *moai*. Explain to your friends the special bond you are committing to and set regular meeting times on the calendar.

12. Volunteer to train a puppy who is preparing to be a service dog.

13. Run a race for a cause that's important to you.

14. Take a yoga, dance, or tai chi class.

15. Join a bird-watching or hiking group.

16. Start a weekly card game with a core group of friends.

17. Join a travel club.

18. Take a plant-based cooking class with a few friends.

19. Start a monthly supper club in which you take turns hosting.

20. Volunteer at your local hospital or homeless shelter.

Journal about any of the above activities that catch your fancy. Then return to your list a few days later and pick three things that feel like they would be beneficial to your life right now. For each of these activities, decide on one small next action you can complete toward making this a reality.

Say yes to the invitation when you are asked to attend, go to the free lecture offered by your public library, or do some research on group meetups in your area. Each time we extend ourselves, we create an opportunity for growth and meaningful connections.

Loving-Kindness Meditation

Loving-kindness meditation is a popular technique to extend forgiveness, kind thoughts, and love to yourself, to others, and to the entire world. This kind of meditation has its origins in Buddhism, where it is called *metta*, a Pali word meaning "loving-kindness, goodwill, and friendliness."

To start, find a spot where you can sit comfortably and be undisturbed for at least ten minutes. Take a few deep breaths and bring your point of focus to the present moment. Try to let all other concerns drop away.

Next, imagine a bright point of glowing, peaceful, beautiful light in your heart. As you breathe, the light expands until it fills your entire body. Sit with this feeling of light and inner peace for a few minutes, and then repeat these positive blessings toward yourself:

May I be happy. May I be at peace. May I be safe. May I be healthy.

(You can change these statements to suit you; just make sure they are positive and uplifting.)

Once you have extended these blessings to yourself, think of someone you're close to—your child or parent, your closest friend—and imagine them also glowing with this peaceful, beautiful inner light. Extend your blessings to them for the next couple of minutes:

May you be happy. May you be at peace. May you be safe. May you be healthy.

Next, think of someone you feel neutral about, like an acquaintance, and while holding them in your mind, continue to expand your blessings outward for the next two to three minutes:

May you be happy. May you be at peace. May you be safe. May you be healthy.

Finally, think of someone you are struggling with or need to forgive—a family member, coworker, or friend with whom you are "out of balance"—and extend the light and blessings to them for the next few minutes:

May you be happy. May you be at peace. May you be safe. May you be healthy.

To end the practice, take a few more deep breaths and open your eyes. You may want to write about your experience in a journal.

I know this last part can be difficult in some circumstances. Be patient, and remind yourself that this forgiveness is for you, not the other person. It takes great courage to even consider doing this in some cases. I salute you.

Ho'oponopono

Oftentimes our relationships can become strained for a variety of reasons over long periods of time. Perhaps there are things we have said or done which we aren't proud of, but a formal apology may not be necessary, helpful, or even possible. In these cases, I invite you to try Ho'oponopono, a practice of reconciliation that comes from the indigenous communities of Hawaii and Polynesia. It has been adapted over time to become a practice of self-forgiveness as well. The word can be translated as "to make right."

At the heart of Ho'oponopono is the recitation of four simple yet powerful phrases—but rather than saying them to the person you have a conflict with, you close your eyes and speak them to yourself while keeping that person in mind.

The phrases are:

I'm sorry. Please forgive me. Thank you. I love you.

While I don't know of any scientific study that has measured why or how this works, I do know this is a practice that has been in place for hundreds, if not thousands, of years. I have a friend who swears by it, and he says it worked in repairing a fractured relationship with a family member when nothing else would. After learning about the practice, he committed to repeating the mantra each evening before he went to bed for ten nights in a row. Over the days that followed, he noticed how each night after repeating those phrases he felt a little better about the conflict. That likely would have been enough for him to say the practice was beneficial, but what happened after that is what really sold him on it. The following week, after not having spoken to this family member in years, she called him just to see how he was doing. My friend said he got chills when he saw her number on his caller ID. He also said that while neither of them discussed their past hurts, the relationship has continued to improve to the point that nothing else really needs to be said.

What I also find interesting about Ho'oponopono is that the ancient peoples who advocated it saw it as medicine, because they felt that holding on to interpersonal conflict could manifest in physical illness. That reminded me of recent studies that have shown how forgiveness can improve your mental and physical health and how anger and hostility can increase your chances of developing coronary heart disease.[18] If you have a relationship that needs to be mended and speaking about the issues directly either isn't possible or might only make the relationship worse, I encourage you to give this powerful practice a try.

Conclusion

In this book, I've shared the turnaround in my own life and the management of my chronic illness through the principles of lifestyle medicine. I credit these changes as the simplest, most direct, and most profound actions for my health and well-being that I have ever undertaken. When I support the adoption of these changes in my patients, colleagues, friends, and family—and now with the readers of this book—I feel a sense of overwhelming pride and hope.

On the difficult days, when I become overwhelmed by the amount of work we have yet to do in the fields of public health, medical education, and health care, I remember one of my favorite stories of societal transformation, which took place over many years in North Karelia, Finland.

In the 1960s, the Finnish people became aware that cardiovascular disease was running rampant and that Finland had the highest rate of coronary heart disease mortality in the world. How did this come to be? After World War II, living standards improved dramatically in Finland, and the dairy industry in particular flourished. Once limited by low production and high cost, people suddenly had the means to eat more dairy products, and consumption skyrocketed. Due to a shorter growing season and less investment in production, fruit and vegetable agriculture did not keep pace. The Finnish diet became rich in butter, cream, whole milk, and cheese, which amounted to a large percentage of saturated fat. Additionally, Finnish veterans returning from the war had picked up a terrible tobacco habit. At its peak, 60 percent of the men were smokers. These factors both played a huge role in Finland's climbing cardiovascular deaths.

In response to this, the Finnish government initiated the North Karelia Project in the 1970s, a vast campaign to inform the public and change the behaviors that were related to heart disease deaths. Newspapers, magazines, radio, and TV were flooded with health-related topics. Health-care professionals and the general community took part in seminars about healthy habits. Locals volunteered to hand out leaflets in their villages. Food service workers in schools, hospitals, and cafeterias received new training.

Things did not change overnight, but the Finns kept going.

The government published dietary guidelines and held a national cholesterol consensus meeting in 1989. Women's organizations held "longevity" or "healthy" parties, where volunteers would give a talk on healthy lifestyle behaviors like not smoking, cutting salt intake, and adding more vegetables to one's diet. During these parties they would share cooking demos and serve healthier, plant-based meals.

Knowing the Finnish people would not readily give up their beloved sausages, government officials convinced local sausage-making businesses to reduce salt and replace pork fat with local mushrooms as a filler. Business leaders were reluctant to do so at first, but they found that when they tried out these new recipes their sales improved. The Finns also realized that they needed to increase consumption of fruit, but imports were pricey. North Karelians only ate the berries that grew locally in the summer months. So the government helped set up ways to freeze and distribute these berries throughout the year. The resulting boost in fruit sales encouraged dairy farmers to section off part of their land to grow more berries.

Over time, the Finnish people grew increasingly aware of the importance of their dietary and lifestyle behaviors, made the investments of time, energy, and money, and followed through on their commitment to better health. These changes resulted in a stunning 73 percent reduction in coronary heart disease mortality in North Karelia specifically and a 65 percent reduction in coronary heart disease mortality in Finland overall from 1972 to 1997.[1]

There is so much we can learn from and be inspired by in the North Karelia story. This powerful example illustrates what can be accomplished when communities work together to achieve a common goal. In order to execute a massive global public health success story of this kind, we all need to come together with a common objective in mind: doctors, patients, communities, cities, states, businesses, and governments. I believe doctors and their patients can lead the way, initiating the first step of awareness on a cultural level.

At the start of this book, we talked about the complicated relationship between medical institutions and the business world, and the financial incentives available to physicians and hospitals that distort the very meaning of "health care." Today, illnesses are treated with drugs and procedures without consideration of the root causes of disease. We must prioritize prevention and lifestyle changes that have overall higher success rates in minimizing symptoms and eradicating disease before it starts.

Under the current system, doctors become highly trained disease detectives, focusing on pathogenesis, or the process of disease. They painstakingly learn how to collect clues to arrive at a diagnosis. They collect information from the patient's history and examination, ordering things like blood work and imaging studies. Once a diagnosis is made, they "solve" the problem by writing a prescription or ordering a surgical procedure.

Meanwhile, medical students and doctors are learning little to nothing about the other end of the human health continuum, which is called salutogenesis. This phrase was coined by Aaron Antonovsky, a professor of medical sociology, in order to "focus on people's resources and capacity to create health rather than the classic focus on risks, ill health, and disease."[2] Salutogenesis is the process by which we produce health and well-being, and according to Dr. David Eisenberg of the Harvard School of Public Health, it "should assume its rightful position alongside the study of pathogenesis . . . in medical education and practice."[3]

When medical schools place salutogenesis on the same level of importance as pathogenesis, we will see a sustainable global shift in the physician role. Doctors will train in modules on nutrition, exercise, stress management, sleep hygiene, substance intake, and social connectedness. Doctors will represent the healthiest amongst us, serving as the example to their patients. The environments in which they practice medicine ought to be representative of optimal health as well. Medical clinics can be stocked with whole foods and healthy snacks, and hospital cafeterias can be powerhouses of nutrition, providing food that prevents disease and maintains health. My hope is that one day we'll marvel at how it could have possibly been any other way, much the same way we are astonished at how at one point in time it was acceptable for doctors to smoke while making rounds in the hospital.

Even if it feels like we have a long way to go in how we view medicine and health, and it's true that many are in denial about what's missing and broken in our system, you have taken the initiative to educate yourself about lifestyle medicine and how it can improve your health and even your whole life in any number of profound ways. You know that the greatest benefits of the lifestyle medicine wheel come through tending to each spoke simultaneously. You will keep learning, and you will keep refining the plan you have put in motion, backing up your successes with more investment and evaluating your failures and trying again. The goal is to live your optimal existence, free of chronic disease and unnecessary pain and suffering. This is your personal journey to optimal health, and you are in control. On a community level, your work will help fuel a shift in the health-care paradigm we so badly need.

The Aha Moment

What triggers a big aha moment that leads to lasting change? For me it was the study on blueberries and MS outcomes I mentioned in the introduction, as this started a search that would end in me making the most significant changes in my life. For other people, it may be an acute, life-altering event like suffering a heart attack or the loss of a loved one. Others may suddenly notice that their clothes always smell like smoke or that they have been struggling with chronic disease and can't stand it one moment longer. Sometimes this moment seems to simply come out of nowhere.

In any case, how is it that we suddenly find it within ourselves to accept the challenge and do what we had never been able to do in the past? This is a difficult question! As a physician, I would give anything to capture this moment so I could recreate it for my patients who are struggling to produce it for themselves.

My best guess is that what we perceive as a singular aha moment is actually an accumulation of smaller events, full of things like awareness, frustration, and inspiration. In other words, rather than an "overnight success," many aha moments might only occur after a steady, lengthy trajectory of building awareness and staying open to what's possible.

I hope this book can be a part of your aha moment.

Acknowledgments

While filming *Code Blue* in 2017, I was offered an opportunity to write a book about my work, but my gut feeling was that something wasn't quite right with the timing and I turned down the offer. But I wondered afterward whether I had made a mistake by doing so. Would an offer ever come again? Did I miss my one chance?

Then, two years later my friend Jay Stinnett encouraged me to pursue writing a book. He added, "I know the perfect person to support you on this creative process, and he also happens to be one of my favorite people on the planet. His name is Randy Davila, and he is the president of Hierophant Publishing."

On May 5, 2019, I met Randy, and I immediately knew it was both the right time and right person. I am forever indebted to Randy for his patience and gentle guidance throughout this journey. Thank you for creating a book that captures my voice and simple essence.

To my husband Ralph, to whom this book is dedicated, I love you more with each passing day. You are the best man I know. Thank you for making all of this possible.

To my children who embody everything I got right: First, to my son Nicholas, thank you for being the one person in the world I know who truly loves everyone unconditionally. To my daughter Emily, whose beautiful voice and immeasurable talent always leave me breathless, thank you for filling my heart with melodious joy.

I want to offer my gratitude to my entire family; both the Stancics and Pellecchias for their support on the home front. I love you all.

To my friend Dilip Barman, who has supported my mission on several fronts to disseminate this health-promoting message, I am so very grateful.

An abundance of gratitude to the extraordinary members of my *moai*; Anne Bertasso, Donna Tarzian, Ken Reinhard, and Kathy Woods, who always encouraged, never doubted, and insisted I forge forward when I was ready to surrender. Thank you for making a lion of this mouse.

Finally, to my loving parents who valiantly immigrated to the United States to offer a better life for their children: Mami y Papi en el cielo; los quiero mucho.

Appendix A: Food Diary Template

Keeping a food journal can be very informative and will help you identify habits—both good and bad. It can also be helpful in determining food allergies or intolerances, as well as imbalances in the diet and possible sources of deficiencies or excess.

For one week, list all the foods and beverages you consume, and take note of the meals eaten at home versus those out. Tips:

- Record everything that crosses your lips! If you are at a restaurant and can't journal at the time, take a photo with your smartphone. Having an image will help you recall what you have consumed later.

- Be as detailed as you can.

- Be sure to include any alcoholic beverages.

I suggest photocopying the chart on the next page and keeping a few copies on hand.

After recording one week's worth of your diet, step back and look at what you've written. See if you can spot any trends, patterns, or habits. For example, you might consider:

- How healthy is my diet?

- Am I eating vegetables and fruit every day?

- Am I eating whole grains each day?

- Have I included legumes into my diet?

- Am I eating foodstuffs?

- How have I reduced animal sources?

- Do my moods affect my eating habits? Do I reach for unhealthy snacks when I'm tired or stressed?

- How often do I eat on the run?

- How often do I eat alone, versus with others?

- How often do I eat out or pick up takeout?

Once you've identified areas for improvement, set one or two healthy eating goals for yourself. See the exercises at the end of chapter 3 for ideas on how to incorporate these insights into a new way of eating.[1]

START DATE	DAY 1	DAY 2	DAY 3	DAY 4	DAY 5	DAY 6	DAY 7
Breakfast							
Time:							
Place:							
Mood:							
Midmorning Snack							
Time:							
Place:							
Mood:							
Lunch							
Time:							
Place:							
Mood:							
Midafternoon Snack							
Time:							
Place:							
Mood:							
Dinner							
Time:							
Place:							
Mood:							
Document all beverages. This should be primarily water.							

Appendix B: Sleep Diary Template

Monitoring your sleep habits is a tool to not only assess your baseline health, but also gauge how incremental changes in other areas of the lifestyle medicine wheel are affecting your sleep, be it diet, exercise, stress management, etc. You may be surprised to find out that making a few small changes, like leaving your smartphone in another room at night, investing in some blackout curtains, and curbing your use of caffeine and alcohol, can make a huge difference in getting to sleep and staying asleep.

Remember, the goal is to get between seven and nine hours of quality sleep every night. I know sometimes this won't be possible, for lots of reasons. The key is to stick to a routine that will encourage healthy habits. What we do *most of the time* matters; the outliers are simply that—outliers.

If, after making some incremental improvements to your sleep routine, you aren't seeing positive results, please talk to your doctor. Something else might be going on, and you'll want to get it checked out.

I suggest photocopying the following two pages and making copies for multiple weeks.

COMPLETE IN THE MORNING							
START DATE	**DAY 1**	**DAY 2**	**DAY 3**	**DAY 4**	**DAY 5**	**DAY 6**	**DAY 7**
I went to bed last night at:	a.m. / p.m.	a.m. / p.m.	a.m. / p.m.	a.m. / p.m.	a.m. / p.m.	a.m. / p.m.	a.m. / p.m.
I woke up this morning at:	a.m. / p.m.	a.m. / p.m.	a.m. / p.m.	a.m. / p.m.	a.m. / p.m.	a.m. / p.m.	a.m. / p.m.
LAST NIGHT I FELL ASLEEP:							
Easily	☐	☐	☐	☐	☐	☐	☐
After Some Time	☐	☐	☐	☐	☐	☐	☐
With Difficulty	☐	☐	☐	☐	☐	☐	☐
I WOKE UP DURING THE NIGHT:							
# of Times							
# of Minutes							
Last night I slept a total of:	hours	hours	hours	hours	hours	hours	hours
MY SLEEP WAS DISTURBED BY: **(E.G., NOISE, LIGHTS, PETS, ALLERGIES, TEMPERATURE, DISCOMFORT, STRESS, ETC.)**							
WHEN I WOKE UP FOR THE DAY, I FELT:							
Refreshed	☐	☐	☐	☐	☐	☐	☐
Somewhat Refreshed	☐	☐	☐	☐	☐	☐	☐
Fatigued	☐	☐	☐	☐	☐	☐	☐
Notes: Record any other factors that may affect your sleep (e.g., work or monthly cycle for women)							

COMPLETE AT THE END OF THE DAY

START DATE	DAY 1	DAY 2	DAY 3	DAY 4	DAY 5	DAY 6	DAY 7
I CONSUMED CAFFEINATED DRINKS IN THE:							
Morning	☐	☐	☐	☐	☐	☐	☐
Afternoon	☐	☐	☐	☐	☐	☐	☐
Evening	☐	☐	☐	☐	☐	☐	☐
N/A	☐	☐	☐	☐	☐	☐	☐
How Many?							
I EXERCISED AT LEAST 30 MINUTES IN THE:							
Morning	☐	☐	☐	☐	☐	☐	☐
Afternoon	☐	☐	☐	☐	☐	☐	☐
Evening	☐	☐	☐	☐	☐	☐	☐
N/A	☐	☐	☐	☐	☐	☐	☐
MEDICATIONS I TOOK TODAY:							
Took a Nap?	Y/N	Y/N	Y/N	Y/N	Y/N	Y/N	Y/N
If yes, for how long?							
How likely was I to doze off while performing daily activies:	No chance / Slight chance / Moderate chance / High chance	No chance / Slight chance / Moderate chance / High chance	No chance / Slight chance / Moderate chance / High chance	No chance / Slight chance / Moderate chance / High chance	No chance / Slight chance / Moderate chance / High chance	No chance / Slight chance / Moderate chance / High chance	No chance / Slight chance / Moderate chance / High chance
During the day, my mood was:	Very pleasant / Pleasant / Unpleasant / Very unpleasant	Very pleasant / Pleasant / Unpleasant / Very unpleasant	Very pleasant / Pleasant / Unpleasant / Very unpleasant	Very pleasant / Pleasant / Unpleasant / Very unpleasant	Very pleasant / Pleasant / Unpleasant / Very unpleasant	Very pleasant / Pleasant / Unpleasant / Very unpleasant	Very pleasant / Pleasant / Unpleasant / Very unpleasant
APPROXIMATELY 2 TO 3 HOURS BEFORE BED, I CONSUMED:							
Alchohol	☐	☐	☐	☐	☐	☐	☐
Nicotine	☐	☐	☐	☐	☐	☐	☐
Caffeine	☐	☐	☐	☐	☐	☐	☐
N/A	☐	☐	☐	☐	☐	☐	☐
IN THE HOUR BEFORE BED, MY ROUTINE INCLUDED: (LIST ACTIVITIES INCLUDING READING A BOOK, USING ELECTRONICS, TAKING A BATH, MEDITATING, JOURNALING, ETC.)							

Notes

Preface

1. Safiya Richardson et al., "Presenting Characteristics, Comorbidities, and Outcomes Among 5700 Patients Hospitalized with COVID-19 in the New York City Area," *JAMA* 323, no. 20 (April 22, 2020): 2052–2059, https://jamanetwork.com/journals/jama/fullarticle/2765184; Erin K. Stokes et al., "Coronavirus Disease 2019 Case Surveillance—United States, January 22–May 30, 2020," *Morbidity and Mortality Weekly Report* 69, no. 24 (June 19, 2020): 759–765, https://www.cdc.gov/mmwr/volumes/69/wr/mm6924e2. htm#suggestedcitation; Grasselli G, Greco M, Zanella A, et al., "Risk Factors Associated With Mortality Among Patients With COVID-19 in Intensive Care Units in Lombardy, Italy," *JAMA Intern Med.* (July 15, 2020), https://jamanetwork.com/journals/jamainternalmedicine/fullarticle/2768601; Sun, Y., Feng, Y., Chen, J., Li, B., Luo, Z., & Wang, P., "Clinical features of fatalities in patients with COVID-19," *Disaster Medicine and Public Health Preparedness* (July 15, 2020): 1–10, https://www.cambridge.org/core/journals/disaster-medicine-and-public-health-preparedness/article/clinical-features-of-fatalities-in-patients-with-covid19/6C0D35474BC11E80D3F6B76F049BA6B7.

2. American Heart Association News, "More Than 100 million Americans Have High Blood Pressure, AHA Says," January 31, 2018, https://www.heart.org/en/news/2018/05/01/more-than-100-million-americans-have-high-blood-pressure-aha-says. Centers for Disease Control and Prevention, "Long-term Trends in Diabetes," https://www.cdc.gov/diabetes/statistics/slides/long_term_trends.pdf; Centers for Disease Control and Prevention, "Adult Obesity Maps," https://www.cdc.gov/obesity/data/prevalence-maps.html.

3. NCD Risk Factor Collaboration, "Trends in Adult Body-Mass Index in 200 Countries from 1975 to 2014: A Pooled Analysis of 1698 Population-Based Measurement Studies with 19.2 Million Participants," *Lancet* 387, no. 10026 (April 2, 2016): 1377–1396, https://www.thelancet.com/journals/lancet/article/PIIS0140-6736(16)30054-X/fulltext.

4. Patti Neighmond, "Overweight People Are More Apt to Ditch Doctors," May 27, 2013, https://www.npr.org/sections/health-shots/2013/05/27/186428233/overweight-people-are-more-apt-to-ditch-doctors.

Introduction

1. R. L. Swank et al., "Multiple Sclerosis in Rural Norway: Its Geographic and Occupational Incidence in Relation to Nutrition," *New England Journal of Medicine* 246 (1952): 721–728.

2. Grytten N, Torkildsen Ø, Myhr KM., "Time trends in the incidence and prevalence of multiple sclerosis in Norway during eight decades," *Acta Neurol Scand* 132, no. S199 (2015): 29–36, https://onlinelibrary.wiley.com/doi/10.1111/ane.12428.

3. R. L. Swank, "Multiple Sclerosis: Twenty Years on Low Fat Diet," *Archives of Neurology* 23, no. 5 (November 1970): 460–474, https://doi.org/10.1001/archneur.1970.00480290080009; R. L. Swank and B. B. Dugan, "Effect of Low Saturated Fat Diet in Early and Late Cases of Multiple Sclerosis," *Lancet* 336, no. 8706 (July 7, 1990): 37–39.

4. P. Ghadirian et al., "Nutritional Factors in the Aetiology of Multiple Sclerosis: A Case-Control Study in Montreal, Canada," *International Journal of Epidemiology* 27, no. 5 (October 1998): 845–852; M. L. Esparza, S. Sasaki, and H. Kesteloot, "Nutrition, Latitude, and Multiple Sclerosis Mortality: An Ecologic Study," *American Journal of Epidemiology* 142, no. 7 (October 1, 1995): 733–737.

Chapter 1: The Man-Made Epidemic of Chronic Disease

1. Centers for Disease Control and Prevention, "Leading Causes of Death, 1900–1998," https://www.cdc.gov/nchs/data/dvs/lead1900_98.pdf.

2. World Health Organization, "Noncommunicable Diseases," June 1, 2018, https://www.who.int/news-room/fact-sheets/detail/noncommunicable-diseases. The WHO defines noncommunicable diseases (NCDs) or

chronic diseases as illnesses of long duration that arise as a consequence of "a combination of genetic, physiological, environmental and behavioral factors."

3. Centers for Disease Control and Prevention, "Table 1. Leading Causes of Death and Numbers of Deaths, by Sex, Race, and Hispanic Origin: United States, 2017," https://www.cdc.gov/nchs/data/nvsr/nvsr68/nvsr68_06-508.pdf.

4. Sherry L. Murphy et al., "Mortality in the United States, 2017," Centers for Disease Control and Prevention, NCHS Data Brief no. 328 (November 2018), https://www.cdc.gov/nchs/data/databriefs/db328-h.pdf. In a recent interview, Dr. C. Michael Valentine, president of the American College of Cardiology, remarked on the frustrating hold of heart disease in the number one spot on the list, noting "Nearly half of all Americans have high blood pressure, high cholesterol or smoke—some of the leading risk factors for heart disease—but these are often either preventable or modifiable risk factors that we can all work to reduce." Richard C. Becker, "CDC: Heart Disease, Cancer Leading Causes of Death in 2017," Healio, November 29, 2018, https://www.healio.com/news/cardiology/20181129/cdc-heart-disease-cancer-leading-causes-of-death-in-2017.

5. CDC's Division of Diabetes Translation, "Long-Term Trends in Diabetes," April 2017, https://www.cdc.gov/diabetes/statistics/slides/long_term_trends.pdf.

6. Centers for Disease Control and Prevention, "National Diabetes Statistics Report, 2020: Estimates of Diabetes and Its Burden in the United States," https://www.cdc.gov/diabetes/pdfs/data/statistics/national-diabetes-statistics-report.pdf; Centers for Disease Control and Prevention, "Number of Americans with Diabetes Projected to Double or Triple by 2050," October 22, 2010, https://www.cdc.gov/media/pressrel/2010/r101022.html.

7. Centers for Disease Control and Prevention, "Health and Economic Costs of Chronic Diseases," https://www.cdc.gov/chronicdisease/about/costs/index.htm.

8. Earl S. Ford et al., "Healthy Living Is the Best Revenge: Findings from the European Prospective Investigation into Cancer and Nutrition–Potsdam Study," *Archives of Internal Medicine* 169, no. 15 (August 10, 2009): 1355–1362.

9. Behavioral Risk Factor Surveillance System, CDC, "2018 BRFSS English Questionnaire," January 18, 2018, https://www.cdc.gov/brfss/questionnaires/pdf-ques/2018_BRFSS_English_Questionnaire.pdf.

10. Centers for Disease Control and Prevention, "Overweight & Obesity: Adult Obesity Maps," October 29, 2019, http://www.cdc.gov/obesity/data/prevalence-maps.html; Centers for Disease Control and Prevention, "Diabetes Growth Rate Steady, Adding to Health Care Burden," July 18, 2017, https://www.cdc.gov/media/releases/2017/p0718-diabetes-report.html.

11. Hales CM, Carroll MD, Fryar CD, Ogden CL. "Prevalence of Obesity and Severe Obesity Among Adults: United States, 2017–2018," *NCHS Data Brief*, no. 360 (2020), https://www.cdc.gov/nchs/data/databriefs/db360-h.pdf.

12. Centers for Disease Control and Prevention, "National Center for Health Statistics: Obesity and Overweight," 2018, https://www.cdc.gov/nchs/fastats/obesity-overweight.htm.

13. Centers for Disease Control and Prevention, "National Center for Chronic Disease Prevention and Health Promotion (NCCDPHP): About Chronic Diseases," October 23, 2019, https://www.cdc.gov/chronicdisease/about/index.htm.

14. Aaron Lerner, Patricia Jeremias, and Torsten Matthias, "The World Incidence and Prevalence of Autoimmune Diseases Is Increasing," *International Journal of Celiac Disease* 3, no. 4 (2015): 151–155; Arndt Manzel et al., "Role of 'Western Diet' in Inflammatory Autoimmune Diseases," *Current Allergy and Asthma Reports* 14, no. 1 (January 2014): 404. Lerner et al. discuss a possible explanation for this startling increase in their paper, saying, "The recent outbreak of autoimmune diseases in industrialized countries has brought into question the factors contributing to this increased incidence. Given the constancy of genetics, growing attention has focused on environmental factors, and in particular, the western lifestyle."

15. Judith M. Greer and Pamela A. McCombe, "The Role of Epigenetic Mechanisms and Processes in Autoimmune Disorders," *Biologics* 6 (2012): 307–327.

16. Manzel et al., "Role of 'Western Diet' in Inflammatory Autoimmune Diseases," 304.

17. David C. Mohr et al., "A Randomized Trial of Stress Management for the Prevention of New Brain Lesions in MS," *Neurology* 79, no. 5 (July 2012): 412–419.

18. Manzel et al., "Role of 'Western Diet' in Inflammatory Autoimmune Diseases," 304.

19. Mark Terry, "Drum Roll, Please! Top 10 Bestselling Drugs in the U.S.," BioSpace, May 21, 2018, https://www.biospace.com/article/drumroll-please-top-10-bestselling-drugs-in-the-u-s-/.

20. Pierce JP, Stefanick ML, Flatt SW, et al., "Greater Survival After Breast Cancer in Physically Active Women with High Vegetable-Fruit Intake Regardless of Obesity," *Journal of Clinical Oncology* 25, no. 17 (June 10, 2007): 2345–2351, https://ascopubs.org/doi/pdf/10.1200/JCO.2006.08.6819.

21. Bria D. Giacomino, Peter Cram, Mary Vaughan-Sarrazin, Yunshu Zhou, and Saket Girotra, "Association of Hospital Prices for Coronary Artery Bypass Grafting with Hospital Quality and Reimbursement," *American Journal of Cardiology* 117, no. 7 (April 2016): 1101–1106, https://doi.org/10.1016/j.amjcard.2016.01.004.

22. Allison Aubrey, "So Long, Big Mac: Cleveland Clinic Ousts McDonald's from Cafeteria," August 19, 2015, https://www.npr.org/sections/thesalt/2015/08/19/432885995/so-long-big-mac-cleveland-clinic-ousts-mcdonalds-from-cafeteria.

23. Eisenberg DM, Burgess JD. "Nutrition Education in an Era of Global Obesity and Diabetes: Thinking Outside the Box," *Academic Medicine* 90, no. 7 (July, 2015): 854–860; Stephen Devries, Walter Willett, and Robert O. Bonow, "Nutrition Education in Medical School, Residency Training, and Practice," *JAMA* 321, no. 14 (April 2019): 1351–1352.

24. M. de Lorgeril et al., "Mediterranean Diet, Traditional Risk Factors, and the Rate of Cardiovascular Complications After Myocardial Infarction: Final Report of the Lyon Diet Heart Study," *Circulation* 99, no. 6 (February 1999): 779–785.

25. William C. Knowler et al., "Reduction in the Incidence of Type 2 Diabetes with Lifestyle Intervention or Metformin," The *New England Journal of Medicine* 346, no. 6 (February 7, 2002): 393–403.

26. Centers for Medicare & Medicaid Services, "The Facts About Open Payments Data: 2018," https://open-paymentsdata.cms.gov/summary.

27. Shahram Ahari, "I Was a Drug Rep. I Know How Pharma Companies Pushed Opioids," *Washington Post*, November 26, 2019, https://www.washingtonpost.com/outlook/i-was-a-drug-rep-i-know-how-pharma-companies-pushed-opioids/2019/11/25/82b1da88-beb9-11e9-9b73-fd3c65ef8f9c_story.html.

28. Jessica Wapner, "How Pharma Changes Your Doctor's Mind," *Newsweek*, May 2, 2017, https://www.newsweek.com/2017/07/14/how-pharma-changes-doctors-minds-593189.html.

29. Ian Larkin et al., "Association Between Academic Medical Center Pharmaceutical Detailing Policies and Physician Prescribing," *JAMA* 317, no. 17 (May 2, 2017): 1785–1795, https://jamanetwork.com/journals/jama/fullarticle/2623607.

Chapter 2: The Lifestyle Medicine Solution

1. National Cancer Institute, "Common Cancer Types," updated February 21, 2019, https://www.cancer.gov/types/common-cancers; Centers for Disease Control and Prevention, "Benefits of Physical Activity," https://www.cdc.gov/physicalactivity/basics/pa-health/index.htm.

2. Debra Blackwell and Tainya Clarke, "State Variation in Meeting the 2008 Federal Guidelines for Both Aerobic and Muscle-Strengthening Activities Through Leisure-Time Physical Activity Among Adults Aged 18–64: United States, 2010–2015," *National Health Statistics Reports* 112, June 28, 2018, https://www.cdc.gov/nchs/data/nhsr/nhsr112.pdf; Centers for Disease Control and Prevention, "Overweight & Obesity: Adult Obesity Maps," October 29, 2019, http://www.cdc.gov/obesity/data/prevalence-maps.html.

3. Allison Soucise et al., "Sleep Quality, Duration, and Breast Cancer Aggressiveness," *Breast Cancer Research and Treatment* 164, no. 1 (July 2017): 169–178, https://doi.org/10.1007/s10549-017-4245-1; David A. Calhoun and Susan M. Harding, "Sleep and Hypertension," *Chest* 138, no. 2 (August 2010): 434–443, https://doi.org/10.1378/chest.09-2954; Ehsan Shokri-Kojori et al., "β-Amyloid Accumulation in the Human Brain

After One Night of Sleep Deprivation," *Proceedings of the National Academy of Sciences,* April 2018, https://doi.org/10.1073/pnas.1721694115.

4. Andressa Alves da Silva et al., "Sleep Duration and Mortality in the Elderly: A Systematic Review with Meta-analysis," *BMJ Open* 6 (February 2016): e008119, https://doi.org/10.1136/bmjopen-2015-008119.

5. Office of Disease Prevention and Health Promotion, "Sleep Health," accessed June 23, 2020, https://www.healthypeople.gov/2020/topics-objectives/topic/sleep-health.

6. U.S. Department of Health and Human Services, *The Health Consequences of Smoking—50 Years of Progress: A Report of the Surgeon General,* Atlanta: U.S. Department of Health and Human Services, Centers for Disease Control and Prevention, National Center for Chronic Disease Prevention and Health Promotion, Office on Smoking and Health, 2014; Office on Smoking and Health, National Center for Chronic Disease Prevention and Health Promotion, "Current Cigarette Smoking Among Adults in the United States," last updated November 18, 2019, https://www.cdc.gov/tobacco/data_statistics/fact_sheets/adult_data/cig_smoking/index.htm.

7. K. Michael Cummings and Robert N. Proctor, "The Changing Public Image of Smoking in the United States: 1964–2014," *Cancer Epidemiology, Biomarkers & Prevention* 23, no. 1 (January 2014): 32–36.

8. Daniel R. Longo et al., "Implementing Smoking Bans in American Hospitals: Results of a National Survey," *Tobacco Control* 7, no. 1 (March 1998): 47–55.

9. Centers for Disease Control and Prevention, "Current Cigarette Smoking Among Adults in the United States," last updated November 18, 2019, https://www.cdc.gov/tobacco/data_statistics/fact_sheets/adult_data/cig_smoking/index.htm.

10. Centers for Disease Control and Prevention, "Fast Facts," last updated May 21, 2020, https://www.cdc.gov/tobacco/data_statistics/fact_sheets/fast_facts/index.htm; Prabhat Jha et al., "21st-Century Hazards of Smoking and Benefits of Cessation in the United States," *New England Journal of Medicine* 368 (2013): 341–350, https://doi.org/10.1056/NEJMsa1211128.

11. Centers for Disease Control and Prevention, "Alcohol Use and Your Health," December 30, 2019, https://www.cdc.gov/alcohol/fact-sheets/alcohol-use.htm.

12. Trisha Petitte et al., "A Systematic Review of Loneliness and Common Chronic Physical Conditions in Adults," *Open Psychology Journal* 8, supplement 2 (2015): 113–132, https://doi.org/10.2174/1874350101508010113.

13. Aislinn Leonard, "Moai—This Tradition Is Why Okinawan People Live Longer, Better," Blue Zones, https://www.bluezones.com/2018/08/moai-this-tradition-is-why-okinawan-people-live-longer-better/.

Chapter 3: The Plant-Centered Plate

1. Michael Pollan, "Unhappy Meals," *New York Times,* January 28, 2007, https://www.nytimes.com/2007/01/28/magazine/28nutritionism.t.html.

2. David A. Kessler, *The End of Overeating: Taking Control of the Insatiable American Appetite* (New York: Rodale, 2009).

3. Alexis Mosca, Marion Leclerc, and Jean P. Hugot, "Gut Microbiota Diversity and Human Diseases: Should We Reintroduce Key Predators in Our Ecosystem?" *Frontiers in Microbiology* 7 (March 2016): 455.

4. Susan V. Lynch and Oluf Pedersen, "The Human Intestinal Microbiome in Health and Disease," *New England Journal of Medicine* 375, no. 24 (December 2016): 2369–2379, https://doi.org/10.1056/NEJMra1600266.

5. Saji, N., Niida, S., Murotani, K. et al. "Analysis of the relationship between the gut microbiome and dementia: a cross-sectional study conducted in Japan." Sci Rep 9, 1008 (2019). https://doi.org/10.1038/s41598-018-38218-7.

6. Mosca A, Leclerc M, Hugot JP, "Gut Microbiota Diversity and Human Diseases: Should We Reintroduce Key Predators in Our Ecosystem?" *Frontiers in Microbiology* 7 (March 31, 2016): 455, https://www.frontiersin.org/articles/10.3389/fmicb.2016.00455/full.

7. Marina Saresella et al., "Immunological and Clinical Effect of Diet Modulation of the Gut Microbiome in Multiple Sclerosis Patients: A Pilot Study," *Frontiers in Immunology* 8 (October 2017): 1391. In this study, a group of MS patients were randomized to either consume a primarily plant-based diet or a Western diet. After a year, stool samples were taken to assess differences in the gut flora. Interestingly, those who ate the plant-enriched diet achieved a diverse gut population with enrichment of a group of organisms called Lachnospiraceae. A significant increase in these bugs is relevant, as they produce positive chemical signals that lead to an anti-inflammatory response. In essence, the presence of this family of microorganisms quieted or cooled down the autoimmune response. Remarkably, the authors concluded relapse rates and disability status were significantly reduced in those who consumed the fiber-rich diet. This and other studies may very well explain how it is a plant-based diet results in improved outcomes in MS patients.

8. Egle Cekanaviciute et al., "Gut Bacteria from Multiple Sclerosis Patients Modulate Human T Cells and Exacerbate Symptoms in Mouse Models," *Proceedings of the National Academy of Sciences* 114, no. 40 (October 3, 2017): 10713–10718.

9. Andrea Maier et al., "Effects of Repeated Exposure on Acceptance of Initially Disliked Vegetables in 7-Month Old Infants," *Food Quality and Preference* 18, no. 8 (December 2007): 1023–1032, https://www.science-direct.com/science/article/abs/pii/S0950329307000523?via percent3Dihub.

10. Huaidong Du et al., "Fresh Fruit Consumption in Relation to Incident Diabetes and Diabetic Vascular Complications: A 7-Y Prospective Study of 0.5 Million Chinese Adults," *PLOS Medicine* 14, no. 4 (April 2017): e1002279.

11. Irene Darmadi-Blackberry et al., "Legumes: The Most Important Dietary Predictor of Survival in Older People of Different Ethnicities," *Asia Pacific Journal of Clinical Nutrition* 13, no. 2 (2004): 217–220.

12. Rebecca S. Mozaffarian et al., "Identifying Whole Grain Foods: A Comparison of Different Approaches for Selecting More Healthful Whole Grain Products," *Public Health Nutrition* 16, no. 12 (December 2013): 2255–2264.

13. David R. Jacobs, Lene Frost Andersen, and Rune Blomhoff, "Whole-Grain Consumption Is Associated with a Reduced Risk of Noncardiovascular, Noncancer Death Attributed to Inflammatory Diseases in the Iowa Women's Health Study," *American Journal of Clinical Nutrition* 85, no. 6 (June 2007): 1606–1614.

14. Sam Kass, "How the Obamas' Pantry Got a Healthyish Makeover," *Bon Appetit*, April 27, 2018, https://www.bonappetit.com/story/sam-kass-obamas-pantry.

15. Rebecca Rupp, "Surviving the Sneaky Psychology of Supermarkets," *National Geographic*, June 14, 2015, https://www.nationalgeographic.com/culture/food/the-plate/2015/06/15/surviving-the-sneaky-psychology-of-supermarkets/.

16 Darshana Thacker, "My $1.50 a Day Challenge: Eating a Plant-Based Diet on an Austere Budget," Forks Over Knives, September 10, 2013, https://www.forksoverknives.com/the-latest/my-1-50-a-day-challenge-eating-a-plant-based-diet-on-an-austere-budget/; Darshana Thacker, "Plant-Based on a Budget: How I Ate Well on $5 a Day," Forks Over Knives, June 24, 2015, https://www.forksoverknives.com/wellness/healthy-food-on-tight-budget/

17. Chana Davis, "Busting the Myth of Incomplete Plant-Based Proteins," *Medium*, August 16, 2018, https://medium.com/tenderlymag/busting-the-myth-of-incomplete-plant-based-proteins-960428e7e91e.

18. Sofia Pineda Ochoa, "Vitamin B12: All Your Questions Answered," Forks Over Knives, November 16, 2017, https://www.forksoverknives.com/wellness/vitamin-b12-questions-answered-2/#gs.7gv6yx.

19. Michael Greger, "Vegan B12 Deficiency: Putting It into Perspective," NutritionFacts.org, August 25, 2011, https://nutritionfacts.org/2011/08/25/vegan-b12-deficiency-putting-it-into-perspective/.

20. Theodore M Brasky, Emily White, and Chi-Ling Chen, "Long-Term, Supplemental, One-Carbon Metabo-lism-Related Vitamin B Use in Relation to Lung Cancer Risk in the Vitamins and Lifestyle (VITAL) Cohort," *Journal of Clinical Oncology* 35, no. 30 (October 2017): 3440–3448.

21. Earl S. Ford et al., "Healthy Living Is the Best Revenge: Findings from the European Prospective Investiga-tion into Cancer and Nutrition–Potsdam Study," *Archives of Internal Medicine* 169, no. 15 (August 10, 2009): 1355–1362; M. J. Stampfer, F. B. Hu, J. E. Manson, E. B. Rimm, and W. C. Willett, "Primary Prevention of

Coronary Heart Disease in Women Through Diet and Lifestyle," *New England Journal of Medicine* 343, no. 1 (July 2000): 16–22, https://doi.org/10.1056/NEJM200007063430103; William C. Knowler et al., "Reduction in the Incidence of Type 2 Diabetes with Lifestyle Intervention or Metformin," *New England Journal of Medicine* 346, no. 6 (February 7, 2002): 393–403.

22. Victor W. Zhong et al., "Associations of Dietary Cholesterol or Egg Consumption with Incident Cardiovascular Disease and Mortality," *JAMA* 321, no. 11 (March 2019): 1081–1095. This recent publication in *JAMA* studied nearly 30,000 adults over close to two decades and concluded that a higher consumption of dietary cholesterol or eggs was significantly associated with an increase in cardiovascular death as well as all-cause mortality.

23. Heaney RP, Weaver CM., "Calcium Absorption from Kale," *American Journal of Clinical Nutrition* 51, no. 4 (April 1990): 656–657, https://academic.oup.com/ajcn/article-abstract/51/4/656/4695196?redirectedFrom =fulltext; Yan Song et al., "Whole Milk Intake Is Associated with Prostate Cancer-Specific Mortality Among U.S. Male Physicians," *Journal of Nutrition* 143, no. 2 (February 2013): 189–196. Although the slice of cheese you just consumed may offer some calcium, it comes with baggage: coronary-artery-clogging saturated fat and cholesterol. Dairy products and milk have been linked to cancer as well. A 2013 publication from the Physicians' Health Study, which followed close to 22,000 male participants for twenty-eight years, concluded those who included 2.5 servings of dairy per day had a 12 percent increase of prostate cancer when compared to those who ate less than half a serving.

Chapter 4: The Importance of Movement Every Day

1. Barbara S. Giesser, "Exercise in the Management of Persons with Multiple Sclerosis, "*Therapeutic Advances in Neurological Disorders* 8, no. 3 (May 2015): 123–130, https://doi.org/10.1177/1756285615576663; J. A. Ponichtera-Mulcare, "Exercise and Multiple Sclerosis," *Medicine & Science in Sports & Exerc*ise 25, no. 4 (April 1993): 451–465; Scott L. Davis, Thad E. Wilson, Andrea T. White, and Elliot M. Frohman, "Thermoregulation in Multiple Sclerosis," *Journal of Applied Physiology* 109, no. 5 (November 2010): 1531–1537, https://doi.org/10.1152/japplphysiol.00460.2010. I'm happy to report that this thinking has largely changed. The majority of doctors treating MS, even in a traditional setting, now recognize the importance of being physically activate for their MS patients and encourage them to do so.

2. "Uhthoff's Syndrome," Multiple Sclerosis News Today, n.d., https://multiplesclerosisnewstoday.com/multiple-sclerosis-symptoms/uhthoffs-syndrome/. According to this source, "As the body temperature rises, the ability of damaged nerves to conduct impulses is reduced. Nerve fibers damaged by MS conduct messages to and from the brain much slower, if at all. An increase in body temperature may cause messages to stop being sent, or to be sent even slower, which makes the symptoms worse until the body temperature returns to normal."

3. J. N. Morris and M. D. Crawford, "Coronary Heart Disease and Physical Activity of Work; Evidence of a National Necropsy Survey," *BMJ* 2, no. 5111 (December 1958): 1485–1496.

4. Lin Yang, et al., "Trends in Sedentary Behavior Among the US Population, 2001–2016," *JAMA* 321, no. 16 (April 2019):1587–1597; 2018 Physical Activity Guidelines Advisory Committee, *2018 Physical Activity Guidelines Advisory Committee Scientific Report*, Washington, DC, Department of Health and Human Services, 2018, https://health.gov/sites/default/files/2019-09/PAG_Advisory_Committee_Report.pdf; Bellettiere J, LaMonte MJ, Evenson KR, et al., "Sedentary behavior and cardiovascular disease in older women: The Objective Physical Activity and Cardiovascular Health (OPACH) Study," *Circulation* 139, no. 8 (February 19, 2019): 1036–1046, https://www.ahajournals.org/doi/10.1161/CIRCULATIONAHA.118.035312.

5. *2018 Physical Activity Guidelines Advisory Committee Scientific Report*, Washington, DC, Department of Health and Human Services, 2018, https://health.gov/sites/default/files/2019-09/PAG_Advisory_Committee_Report.pdf.

6. In 2007, the American Medical Association partnered with the American College of Sports Medicine to create a program called Exercise in Medicine, which promotes physical activity and offers both patients and health-care professionals tools to support meeting exercise guidelines. One of the recommendations they offer is actually writing patients a prescription for exercise using the acronym FITT (frequency, intensity, type, time).

7. Twig Mowatt, "Get Healthy, Get a Dog," The Bark, June 2015, https://thebark.com/content/get-healthy-get-dog.

8. Andrea Beetz, Kerstin Uvnäs-Moberg, Henri Julius, and Kurt Kotrschal, "Psychosocial and Psychophysiological Effects of Human-Animal Interactions: The Possible Role of Oxytocin," *Frontiers in Psychology* 3 (July

2012): 234, https://doi.org/10.3389/fpsyg.2012.00234; J. K. Vormbrock and J. M. Grossberg, "Cardiovascular Effects of Human-Pet Dog Interactions," *Journal of Behavioral Medicine* 11, no. 5 (October 1988): 509–517, https://doi.org/10.1007/BF00844843.

9. National Center for Complementary and Integrative Health, "Yoga: What You Need to Know," U.S. Department of Health and Human Services, updated May 2019, https://www.nccih.nih.gov/health/yoga-what-you-need-to-know; Harvard Health Publishing, "Yoga for Anxiety and Depression," https://www.health.harvard.edu/mind-and-mood/yoga-for-anxiety-and-depression; Harvard Health Publishing, "Yoga for Better Sleep," https://www.health.harvard.edu/blog/8753-201512048753

10. Mark Hamer and Yoichi Chida, "Active Commuting and Cardiovascular Risk: A Meta-Analytic Review," *Preventive Medicine* 46, no. 1 (January 2008): 9–13.

Chapter 5: Living Better with Mindful Stress Management

1. Viktor E. Frankl, *Man's Search for Meaning* (Boston: Beacon Press, 2006).

2. Jeongok G. Logan and Debra J. Bardsdale, "Allostasis and Allostatic Load: Expanding the Discourse on Stress and Cardiovascular Disease," *Journal of Clinical Nursing* 17, no. 7b (July 2008): 201–208. See also Shuji Uchiyama et al., "Job Strain and Risk of Cardiovascular Events in Treated Hypertensive Japanese Workers: Hypertension Follow-Up Group Study," *Journal of Occupational Health* 47, no. 2 (March 2005): 102–111; Chantal Guimont et al., "Effects of Job Strain on Blood Pressure: A Prospective Study of Male and Female White-Collar Workers," *American Journal of Public Health* 96, no. 8 (August 2006): 1436–1443; and P. Armario et al., "Blood Pressure Reactivity to Mental Stress Task as a Determinant of Sustained Hypertension After 5 Years of Follow-Up," *Journal of Human Hypertension* 17, no. 3 (March 2003): 181–186.

3. Bruce S. McEwen and Peter J. Gianaros, "Central Role of the Brain in Stress and Adaptation: Links to Socioeconomic Status, Health, and Disease," *Annals of the New York Academy of Sciences* 1186 (February 2010): 190–222.

4. Bremner JD., "Neuroimaging in Posttraumatic Stress Disorder and Other Stress-Related Disorders," *Neuroimaging Clinics of North America* 17, no. 4 (October 31, 2007): 523-ix, http://europepmc.org/article/MED/17983968; McEwen BS., "Protective and Damaging Effects of Stress Mediators: Central Role of the Brain," *Dialogues in Clinical Neuroscience* 8, no. 4 (December, 2006): 367–381, https://www.ncbi.nlm.nih.gov/pmc/articles/PMC3181832/.

5. B. S. McEwen, "Protective and Damaging Effects of Stress Mediators," *New England Journal of Medicine* 338, no. 3 (January 1998): 171–179.

6. Rapoliene, Lolita, Razbadauskas, Arturas & Jurgelėnas, Antanas. "The Reduction of Distress Using Therapeutic Geothermal Water Procedures in a Randomized Controlled Clinical Trial," *Advances in Preventive Medicine*, (2015), https://www.ncbi.nlm.nih.gov/pmc/articles/PMC4383502/stress response curve adapted from Nixon P: Practitioner (1979); Robert M. Yerkes and John D. Dodson, "The Relation of Strength of Stimulus to Rapidity of Habit-Formation," *Journal of Comparative Neurology and Psychology* 18, no. 5 (November 1908): 459–482.

7. "What is Neuroplasticity?" Psychology Today, https://www.psychologytoday.com/us/basics/neuroplasticity. Neuroplasticity is the capacity of nerve cells to biologically adapt to circumstances—to respond to stimulation by generating new tendrils of connection (synapses) to other nerve cells, and to respond to deprivation and excess stress by weakening connections.

8. Jun S. Lai et al., "A Systematic Review and Meta-analysis of Dietary Patterns and Depression in Community-Dwelling Adults," *American Journal of Clinical Nutrition* 99 no. 1 (January 2014): 181–197.

9. Heather M. Francis et al., "A Brief Diet Intervention Can Reduce Symptoms of Depression in Young Adults—A Randomised Controlled Trial," *PLOS ONE* 14, no. 10 (October 2019): e0222768, https://doi.org/10.1371/journal.pone.0222768.

10. Tobias Esch and George B. Stefano, "Endogenous Reward Mechanisms and Their Importance in Stress Reduction, Exercise and the Brain," *Archives of Medical Science* 6, no. 3 (June 2010): 447–455.

11. Madhav Goyal et al., "Meditation Programs for Psychological Stress and Well-Being: A Systematic Review and Meta-analysis," *JAMA Internal Medicine* 174 no. 3 (March 2014): 357–368, https://doi.org/10.1001/

jamainternmed.2013.13018. Often my colleagues in clinical medicine will question the validity of meditation in Western medicine, suggesting that there is no clear scientific evidence that it offers any true benefit. But researchers at Johns Hopkins University reviewed 47 studies that addressed meditation in patient care and concluded that the practice of meditation can result in as much as "moderate reductions of multiple negative dimensions of psychological stress." Meditation is "medicine," and it should be part of a comprehensive stress-reducing intervention.

12. Robert A. Emmons and Michael E. McCullough, "Counting Blessings Versus Burdens: An Experimental Investigation of Gratitude and Subjective Well-Being in Daily Life," *Journal of Personality and Social Psychology* 84, no. 2 (2003): 377–389, https://greatergood.berkeley.edu/pdfs/GratitudePDFs/6Emmons-BlessingsBurdens.pdf.

Chapter 6: Establishing Good Sleeping Habits

1. National Sleep Foundation, "The Relationship Between Sleep and Industrial Accidents," SleepFoundation. org, https://www.sleepfoundation.org/excessive-sleepiness/safety/relationship-between-sleep-and-industrial-accidents; Daniel J. Gottlieb, Jeffrey M. Ellenbogen, Matt T. Bianchi, and Charles A. Czeisler, "Sleep Deficiency and Motor Vehicle Crash Risk in the General Population: A Prospective Cohort Study," *BMC Medicine* 16, no. 1 (March 2018): 44, https://doi.org/10.1186/s12916-018-1025-7; Charles A. Czeisler, "Impact of Sleepiness and Sleep Deficiency on Public Health—Utility of Biomarkers," *Journal of Clinical Sleep Medicine* 7, no. 5 (October 2011): S6–S8, https://doi.org/10.5664/JCSM.1340; Jason P. Sullivan et al., "Randomized, Prospective Study of the Impact of a Sleep Health Program on Firefighter Injury and Disability," *Sleep* 40, no. 1 (January 2017): zsw001, https://doi.org/10.1093/sleep/zsw001.

2. Kristen L. Knutson, Armand M. Ryden, Bryce A. Mander, and Eve Van Cauter, "Role of Sleep Duration and Quality in the Risk and Severity of Type 2 Diabetes Mellitus," *Archives of Internal Medicine* 166, no. 16 (September 2006): 1768–1774, https://doi.org/10.1001/archinte.166.16.1768.

3. National Heart, Lung, and Blood Institute, "Your Guide to Healthy Sleep," https://www.nhlbi.nih.gov/health-topics/all-publications-and-resources/your-guide-healthy-sleep; Centers for Disease Control and Prevention, "Sleep and Chronic Disease," https://www.cdc.gov/sleep/about_sleep/chronic_disease.html; American Sleep Association, "REM Sleep: Why is it important?" https://www.sleepassociation.org/about-sleep/stages-of-sleep/rem-sleep/.

4. Williamson AM, Feyer AM. "Moderate Sleep Deprivation Produces Impairments in Cognitive and Motor Performance Equivalent to Legally Prescribed Levels of Alcohol Intoxication," *Occupational and Environmental Medicine* 57, no. 10 (October 1, 2000): 649–655, https://oem.bmj.com/content/57/10.

5. Division of Nutrition, Physical Activity, and Obesity, National Center for Chronic Disease Prevention and Health Promotion, "Adult Obesity Facts," CDC, reviewed February 27, 2020, https://www.cdc.gov/obesity/data/adult.html; Spicuzza L, Caruso D, Di Maria G., "Obstructive Sleep Apnoea Syndrome and Its Management," *Therapeutic Advances in Chronic Disease* 6, no. 5 (July 9, 2015): 273–285, https://journals.sagepub.com/doi/10.1177/2040622315590318.

6. Merrill M. Mitler et al., "Catastrophes, Sleep, and Public Policy: Consensus Report," *Sleep* 11, no. 1: 100–109, https://doi.org/10.1093/sleep/11.1.100.

7. E. Kasasbeh, David S. Chi, and G. Krishnaswamy, "Inflammatory Aspects of Sleep Apnea and Their Cardiovascular Consequences," *Southern Medical Journal* 99, no. 1 (January 2006): 58–67; S. Taheri, "The Link Between Short Sleep Duration and Obesity: We Should Recommend More Sleep to Prevent Obesity," *Archives of Disease in Childhood* 91, no. 11 (November 2006): 881–884; Mark Zimmerman et al., "Diagnosing Major Depressive Disorder I: A Psychometric Evaluation of the DSM-IV Symptom Criteria," *Journal of Nervous and Mental Disease* 194, no. 3 (March 2006): 158–163.

8. Thomas C. Erren et al., "Shift Work and Cancer: The Evidence and the Challenge," *Deutsches Ärzteblatt International* 107, no. 38 (September 2010): 657–662, https://doi.org/10.3238/arztebl.2010.0657.

9. Florence Menegaux et al., "Night Work and Breast Cancer: A Population-Based Case–Control Study in France (The CECILE Study)," *International Journal of Cancer* 132, no. 4 (February 2013): 924–931. See also Fangyi Gu et al., "Total and Cause-Specific Mortality of U.S. Nurses Working Rotating Night Shifts," *American Journal of Preventive Medicine* 48, no. 3 (March 2015): 241–252, https://doi.org/10.1016/j.amepre.2014.10.018; Kurt Straif et al., "Carcinogenicity of Shift-Work, Painting, and Fire-Fighting," *Lancet Oncology* 8, no. 12 (December 2007): 1065–1066. These alarming statistics were further bolstered in October 2007 when the

World Health Organization brought international attention to this matter by classifying night shift work as a probable carcinogen due to its disturbance of normal circadian rhythm or what they termed chronodisruption.

10. A. Brzezinski, "Melatonin in Humans," *New England Journal of Medicine* 336, no. 3 (January 1997): 186–195, https://doi.org/10.1056/NEJM199701163360306.

11. D. Léger, B. Poursain, D. Neubauer, and M. Uchiyama, "An International Survey of Sleeping Problems in the General Population," *Current Medical Research and Opinion* 24, no. 1 (January 2008): 307–317, https://doi.org/10.1185/030079907x253771.

12. "Sleep Hygiene," National Sleep Foundation, https://www.sleepfoundation.org/articles/sleep-hygiene.

13. Lisa Ostrin, "Ocular and Systemic Melatonin and the Influence of Light Exposure," *Clinical and Experimental Optometry* 102, no. 2 (August 3, 2018): 99–108, https://pubmed.ncbi.nlm.nih.gov/30074278/.

14. The Sleep Council, "How Much Sleep Do We Need?" https://sleepcouncil.org.uk/advice-support/sleep-hub/sleep-matters/how-much-sleep-do-we-need/.

15. Gustavo Angarita, Nazli Emadi, Sarah Hodges, and Peter T. Morgan, "Sleep Abnormalities Associated with Alcohol, Cannabis, Cocaine, and Opiate Use: A Comprehensive Review," *Addiction Science & Clinical Practice* 11, no. 1 (April 2016): 9, https://doi.org/10.1186/s13722-016-0056-7.

16. Alena Hall, "6 Ways Smoking Affects Your Sleep," HuffPost, March 5, 2015, https://www.huffpost.com/entry/how-smoking-affects-sleep_n_6792954.

17. Matthew A. Christensen et al., "Direct Measurements of Smartphone Screen-Time: Relationships with Demographics and Sleep," *PLOS ONE* 11, no. 11 (November 2016): e0165331, https://doi.org/10.1371/journal.Pone.0165331.

Chapter 7: Substance Intake Awareness

1. E. J. Khantzian, "The Self-Medication Hypothesis of Addictive Disorders," *American Journal of Psychiatry* 142, no. 11 (November 1985): 1259–1264, https://doi.org/10.1176/ajp.142.11.1259.

2. Office on Smoking and Health, National Center for Chronic Disease Prevention and Health Promotion, "Smoking & Tobacco Use," CDC, reviewed November 15, 2019, https://www.cdc.gov/tobacco/data_statistics/fact_sheets/index.htm; Centers for Disease Control and Prevention, "Achievements in Public Health, 1900-1999: Tobacco Use – United States, 1900-1999," https://www.cdc.gov/mmwr/preview/mmwrhtml/mm4843a2.htm.

3. World Health Organization, "Tobacco," May 27, 2020, https://www.who.int/news-room/fact-sheets/detail/tobacco; Our World in Data, "Smoking," https://ourworldindata.org/smoking.

4. Centers for Disease Control and Prevention, "Smoking and Tobacco Use: Cigarette Smoking and Tobacco Use Among People of Low Socioeconomic Status," https://www.cdc.gov/tobacco/disparities/low-ses/index.htm; The Global Adult Tobacco Survey Atlas, http://gatsatlas.org.

5. "Is Drinking Alcohol Part of a Healthy Lifestyle?" American Heart Association, updated December 30, 2019, https://www.heart.org/en/healthy-living/healthy-eating/eat-smart/nutrition-basics/alcohol-and-heart-health.

6. Roxanne Nelson, "American Cancer Society Update: 'It Is Best Not to Drink Alcohol,'" Medscape, June 9, 2020, https://www.medscape.com/viewarticle/931995; L. Rock, Cynthia Thompson, Ted Gansler et al., "American Cancer Society Guidelines for Diet and Physical Activity for Cancer Prevention", *CA: A Cancer Journal for Clinicians* (June 9, 2020): 1–27.

7. Division of Population Health, National Center for Chronic Disease Prevention and Health Promotion, and Centers for Disease Control and Prevention, "Alcohol Use and Your Health," CDC, reviewed December 30, 2019, https://www.cdc.gov/alcohol/fact-sheets/alcohol-use.htm.

8. David W. Baker, "The Joint Commission's Pain Standards: Origins and Evolution," Oakbrook Terrace, IL: The Joint Commission, 2017, https://www.jointcommission.org/-/media/tjc/documents/resources/pain-

management/pain_std_history_web_version_05122017pdf.pdf?db=web&hash=E7D12A5C3BE9DF031F 3D8FE0D8509580.

9. "The Opioid Epidemic by the Number," HHS.gov, updated October 2019, https://www.hhs.gov/opioids/ sites/default/files/2019-11/Opioids%20Infographic_letterSizePDF_10-02-19.pdf.

10. Office on Smoking and Health, National Center for Chronic Disease Prevention and Health Promotion, "Smoking & Tobacco Use: Benefits of Quitting," CDC, reviewed April 28, 2020, https://www.cdc.gov/ tobacco/quit_smoking/how_to_quit/benefits/index.htm.

Chapter 8: The Healing Power of Human Connection

1. CNN, "The Hug That Helped Change Medicine," February 22, 2013, https://www.youtube.com/ watch?v=0YwT_Gx49os.

2. Debra Umberson and Jennifer Karas Montez, "Social Relationships and Health: A Flashpoint for Health Policy," *Journal of Health and Social Behavior* 51 (2010): S54–S66, https://doi.org/10.1177/0022146510383501.

3. William C. Cockerham, Bryant W. Hamby, and Gabriela R. Oates, "The Social Determinants of Chronic Disease," *American Journal of Preventive Medicine* 52, no. 1 supplement 1 (January 2017): S5–S12, https://doi. org/10.1016/j.amepre.2016.09.010; Yang Claire Yang, Kristen Schorpp, and Kathleen Mullan Harris, "Social Support, Social Strain and Inflammation: Evidence from a National Longitudinal Study of U.S. Adults," *Social Science & Medicine* 107 (April 2014): 124–135, https://doi.org/10.1016/j.socscimed.2014.02.013.

4. Yang Claire Yang, Ting Li, and Yinchun Ji, "Impact of Social Integration on Metabolic Functions: Evidence from a Nationally Representative Longitudinal Study of US Older Adults," *BMC Public Health* 13 (December 2013): 1210, https://doi.org/10.1186/1471-2458-13-1210.

5. Sandra D. Bot, Joreintje D. Mackenbach, Giel Nijpels, and Jeroen Lakerveld, "Association Between Social Network Characteristics and Lifestyle Behaviours in Adults at Risk of Diabetes and Cardiovascular Disease," *PLOS ONE* 11, no. 10 (October 2016): e0165041, https://doi.org/10.1371/journal.pone.0165041.

6. Karen A. Ertel, M. Maria Glymour, and Lisa F. Berkman, "Effects of Social Integration on Preserving Memory Function in a Nationally Representative US Elderly Population," *American Journal of Public Health* 98, no. 7 (July 2008): 1215–1220, https://doi.org/10.2105/AJPH.2007.113654.

7. Candyce H. Kroenke et al., "Post-diagnosis Social Networks and Breast Cancer Mortality in the After Breast Cancer Pooling Project (ABCPP)," *Cancer* 123, no. 7 (April 2017): 1228–1237, https://doi. org/10.1002/cncr.30440; Kaiser Permanente, "Women with More Social Connections Have Higher Breast Cancer Survival, Study Shows," Science Daily, December 13, 2016, https://www.sciencedaily.com/ releases/2016/12/161213115055.htm.

8. Christian Hakulinen, Laura Pulkki-Råback, Marianna Virtanen, Markus Jokela, Mika Kivimäki, and Marko Elovainio, "Social Isolation and Loneliness as Risk Factors for Myocardial Infarction, Stroke and Mortality: UK Biobank Cohort Study of 479 054 Men and Women," *Heart* 104, no. 18 (September 2018): 1536–1542, https://doi.org/10.1136/heartjnl-2017-312663.

9. Julianne Holt-Lunstad, Timothy B. Smith, Mark Baker, Tyler Harris, and David Stephenson, "Loneliness and Social Isolation as Risk Factors for Mortality: A Meta-analytic Review," *Perspectives on Psychological Science* 10, no. 2 (March 2015): 227–237, https://doi.org/10.1177/1745691614568352; Timothy P. Daaleman, "The Long Loneliness of Primary Care," *Annals of Family Medicine* 16, no. 5 (September 2018): 388–389, https://doi. org/10.1370/afm.2301.

10. Greater Good Magazine, "Why Practice It?" Greater Good Science Center at UC Berkeley, accessed June 12, 2020, https://greatergood.berkeley.edu/topic/social_connection/definition#why-practice-social-connection.

11. Centers for Disease Control and Prevention, "The State of Aging & Health in America 2013," US Department of Health and Human Services, 2013, https://www.cdc.gov/aging/pdf/state-aging-health-in-america-2013.pdf.

12. Dan Buettner and Sam Skemp, "Blue Zones: Lessons From the World's Longest Lived," *American Journal of Lifestyle Medicine* 10, no. 5 (July 2016): 318–321, https://doi.org/10.1177/1559827616637066.

13. Merriam-Webster, "American dream," accessed June 12, 2020, https://www.merriam-webster.com/dictionary/American percent20dream.

14. Clive Thompson, "Are Your Friends Making You Fat?" *New York Times*, September 10, 2009, https://www.nytimes.com/2009/09/13/magazine/13contagion-t.html.

15. Nicholas A. Christakis and James H. Fowler, "The Spread of Obesity in a Large Social Network over 32 Years," *New England Journal of Medicine* 357 (July 2007): 370–379, https://doi.org/10.1056/NEJMsa066082; Nicholas Christakis, "The Hidden Influence of Social Networks," Ted.com, February 2010, https://www.ted.com/talks/nicholas_christakis_the_hidden_influence_of_social_networks.

16. Fred Rogers, *The World According to Mister Rogers: Important Things to Remember* (New York: Hachette, 2019); John Pattison, "Why Mister Rogers Is More Relevant than Ever," November 21, 2019, https://www.strongtowns.org/journal/2019/11/21/why-mister-rogers-is-more-relevant-than-ever.

17. National Center for Chronic Disease Prevention and Health Promotion, Division of Population Health, "Are You Engaged?" CDC Features, reviewed May 8, 2017, https://www.cdc.gov/features/social-engagement-aging/index.html.

18. Kirsten Weir, "Forgiveness Can Improve Mental and Physical Health," *American Psychological Association*, https://www.apa.org/monitor/2017/01/ce-corner; Yoichi Chida and Andrew Steptoe, "The Association of Anger and Hostility with Future Coronary Heart Disease: A Meta-analytic Review of Prospective Evidence," *Journal of the American College of Cardiology* 53, no. 11 (March 2009): 936–946, https://doi.org/10.1016/j.jacc.2008.11.044.

Conclusion

1. Pekka Puska, "North Karelia Project," University of Minnesota, updated October 15, 2012, http://www.epi.umn.edu/cvdepi/study-synopsis/north-karelia-project/.

2. Wayne B. Jonas, Ronald A. Chez, Katherine Smith, and Bonnie Sakallaris, "Salutogenesis: The Defining Concept for a New Healthcare System," *Global Advances in Health and Medicine* 3, no. 3 (May 2014): 82–91, https://doi.org/10.7453/gahmj.2014.005.

3. David M. Eisenberg and Jonathan D. Burgess, "Nutrition Education in an Era of Global Obesity and Diabetes: Thinking Outside the Box," *Academic Medicine* 90, no. 7 (July 2015): 854–860, https://doi.org/10.1097/ACM.0000000000000682.

Appendix A

1. Components of the food diary were informed by Katherine D. McManus, "Why Keep a Food Diary?" Harvard Health Blog, January 31, 2019, https://www.health.harvard.edu/blog/why-keep-a-food-diary-2019013115855.

About the Author

Saray Stancic, MD is a board-certified physician and the subject of the recent documentary film *Code Blue*.

From 1999 to 2006, Dr. Stancic served as chief of infectious diseases at the Hudson Valley Veterans Administration Hospital in New York. During those years she treated hundreds of patients with viral hepatitis and HIV and directed the MOVE program, a federal VA initiative to encourage healthy lifestyles in veterans.

She later joined the viral hepatology team at Roche and conducted clinical studies for new, more efficacious treatments for hepatitis infections. During these research years, she continued to see patients at the Bronx Veterans Administration Hospital in New York City.

In 2012, in response to her personal experiences as a multiple sclerosis patient as well as a veteran physician, Dr. Stancic founded one of the first lifestyle medicine practices in the country, where she created a distinct contemporary health-care model rooted in traditional medical principles. Dr. Stancic's current practice focuses on educating and empowering patients to understand the importance of the personal lifestyle choices discussed in this book. She mentors medical students and residents and seeks to contribute to initiatives centered on redefining the health-care paradigm. She is a fellow of the American College of Lifestyle Medicine.

Visit her at https://drstancic.com/.

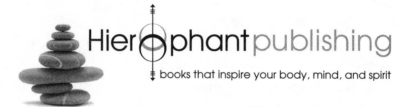

Hierophant Publishing
8301 Broadway, Suite 219
San Antonio, TX 78209
888-800-4240

www.hierophantpublishing.com